THE CRAFT OF EDITING

The Craft of Editing offers a rare insight into the unique dynamic between author and editor. In this illuminating book, Adnan Mahmutović and Lucy Durneen lead a cohort of industry experts to bring transparency to the mystique that often surrounds the craft and practice of editing. Using genuine case studies from published works – including annotated manuscripts – this book prepares writers for potential dialogue and critique from editors. *The Craft of Editing* follows the journey from rough draft to publication, an essential part of any writing experience, while showing the singular and authentic approach each editor takes. Using original pitches, debates, emails, and instant messages to shed light on the collaboration between authors and editors, *The Craft of Editing* is an indispensable tool to creative writers and students alike.

Adnan Mahmutović is Lecturer in English Literature and Creative Writing at the Department of English, Stockholm University, Sweden. He has also been fiction editor at *Two Thirds North*, a journal of transnational writing, since 2010.

Lucy Durneen is Teaching Associate at the Institute of Continuing Education, Cambridge University, UK. Her fiction has been widely published in a collection, *Wild Gestures*, which won the award for Best Short Stories at the 2017 Saboteur Awards, and was longlisted for the 2018 Edge Hill Prize.

THE CRAFT OF EDITING

*Edited by Adnan Mahmutović
and Lucy Durneen*

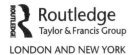

Routledge
Taylor & Francis Group

LONDON AND NEW YORK

First published 2019
by Routledge
2 Park Square, Milton Park, Abingdon, Oxon OX14 4RN

and by Routledge
711 Third Avenue, New York, NY 10017

Routledge is an imprint of the Taylor & Francis Group, an informa business

British Library Cataloguing-in-Publication Data
A catalogue record for this book is available from the British Library

Library of Congress Cataloging-in-Publication Data
Names: Mahmutović, Adnan, editor. | Durneen, Lucy, editor.
Title: The craft of editing / edited by Adnan Mahmutović
and Lucy Durneen.
Description: Milton Park, Abingdon, Oxon; New York,
NY: Routledge, 2018.
Identifiers: LCCN 2018008435 | ISBN 9781138495791
(hardback; alk. paper) | ISBN 9781138495807 (pbk.; alk. paper) |
ISBN 9780429957178 (web) | ISBN 9780429957154 (mobikindle)
Subjects: LCSH: Editing.
Classification: LCC PN162.C69 2018 | DDC 808.02/7–dc23
LC record available at https://lccn.loc.gov/2018008435

ISBN: 978-1-138-49579-1 (hbk)
ISBN: 978-1-138-49580-7 (pbk)
ISBN: 978-0-429-49119-1 (ebk)

Typeset in Bembo
by Sunrise Setting Ltd, Brixham, UK

Printed and bound by CPI Group (UK) Ltd, Croydon, CR0 4YY

CONTENTS

CONTRIBUTORS

Sybil Baker is the author of three books of fiction, *Into This World*, *Talismans*, and *The Life Plan*, and creative non-fiction *Immigration Essays*. She is a 2012 and 2014 MakeWork grantee and received a Tennessee Arts Commission Individual Artist Fellowship for 2017. She is on faculty at the Yale Writers Conference and is Fiction Editor at *Drunken Boat*.

Anna Crofts first had a career as a professional musician (Gothenburg Opera Orchestra). After studies in linguistics and literature (MA in English literature, Stockholm University) she has now been working as a translator and editor for several years.

Jennifer Alise Drew is the nonfiction editor for *AGNI* magazine and has worked as an editor for numerous other magazines and publishers, including *Open City* and *Madison* magazines, *The Huffington Post*, Simon & Schuster, Houghton Mifflin, Grove Atlantic, Aperture, and Open City Books. For a big little while, spanning two books and the last four years of his life, she was a friend and editor to Hunter S. Thompson. She is currently completing a memoir in essays, excerpts from which have appeared in *Slice*, *The Iowa Review*, *The Chattahoochee Review*, *Hippocampus Magazine*, and *Lumina*.

Lucy Durneen is Teaching Associate in Creative Writing at the Institute of Continuing Education, University of Cambridge. Her short stories, poetry, and non-fiction have been published and commended internationally, in journals including *World Literature Today*, *Hotel Amerika*, and *The Amorist*. Her fiction has been Pushcart Prize nominated and Highly Commended in the Manchester Fiction Prize, while her non-fiction has been adapted for broadcast on BBC Radio 4, and listed as a Notable Essay in Best American Essays 2017. Her first short story collection, *Wild Gestures*, was published in 2017, and won Best Short Story Collection at the Saboteur Awards in London in May of the same year.

Robin Hemley is the winner of a Guggenheim Fellowship and many other awards, including the Nelson Algren Award for Fiction from *The Chicago Tribune*, and three Pushcart Prizes. He has published 11 books and his stories and essays have appeared in the *New York Times*, *New York Magazine*, *Chicago Tribune*, and many literary magazines and anthologies. Robin directed the Nonfiction Writing Program at The University of Iowa for nine years. He is currently Writer-in-Residence and Director of the Writing Program at Yale-NUS in Singapore.

Friðrik Sólnes Jónsson is an Icelandic electrician living in Stockholm. Friðrik holds an MA in literature in English and has had stories published by The Wales Art Review, Short Fiction Journal and Two Thirds North. Friðrik has also written prologues for books by comic artist Hugleikur Dagsson, fifteen in all, and writes regular book reviews for the Icelandic online cultural journal Starafugl.

Adnan Mahmutović is a Bosnian-Swedish writer and lecturer at Stockholm University. His works include *Visions of the Future in Comics* (McFarland Press, 2017), *Ways of Being Free* (Rodopi, 2010), *Thinner than a Hair* (Cinnamon Press, 2010), *How to Fare Well and Stay Fair* (Salt Publishing, 2012). He leads an MA in Transnational Creative Writing at Stockholm University.

Vince Passaro is the author of *Violence, Nudity, Adult Content: A Novel* (Simon and Schuster, 2002), and is currently at work on a second book of fiction. His work has appeared in *Harper's Magazine*, where he is a contributing editor, *Esquire*, *GQ*, *The New York Times Sunday Magazine*, *The New York Times Book Review*, *Story*, *Boulevard*, *Open City*, and *AGNI*. He blogs at *Bitter Conceits*.

Jennifer Sahn is Executive Editor of *Pacific Standard*. She previously served as Editor of *Orion*, during which time the magazine was twice a winner of the Utne Independent Press Award for General Excellence and twice a finalist for a National Magazine Award. She has been a judge for several literary awards and fellowships. Stories she has edited have been awarded the Pushcart Prize, O. Henry Prize, John Burroughs Essay Award, and have been widely reprinted in the Best American Series anthologies, *The Norton Reader*, and via online aggregators such as Longreads.

Autumn Watts, Fiction Editor of *Guernica*, has an MFA in fiction from Cornell, and lives in Ankara, Turkey. Her work has appeared in *Guernica*, *AGNI Online*, and *Indiana Review*, among others, and she is the co-editor of *Constructing Qatar: Migrant Narratives From the Margins of a Global System*. She is currently finishing a collection of oral Qatari folktales.

1

THE CRAFT OF EDITING

Adnan Mahmutović and Lucy Durneen

A truism. All writers need editors.

— *Blake Morrison (2005)*

There is no doubt that editing is essential to writing, but the aim of the volume before you is to ask not only what is essential to editing but most importantly, how might we study editing as a craft?

As in any field, there are many books which deal with theoretical aspects and there are few which actually show how something is practiced. A typical book on editing might explain some principles and show examples of elements such as editing for content, editing for grammar, editing for flow, editing for style, etc. While valuable, such books will not give much insight into the complex realities of the editing processes, whether to a novice or a more experienced writer. For this reason, this volume presents real cases which show texts being shaped and transformed into polished, published, and praised works. You will see how much relationships between, and attitudes of authors and editors affect the finished text. You will have access to the behind-the-scenes materials not available anywhere else. While all the cases will contain recognisable elements that are common to all editing processes, each separate case shows how elements like editing for language can be very individual. This book is aimed at higher level students of creative writing, from graduate students of MAs and MFAs to experienced writers. While students with little experience will no doubt find it useful because they will be reading less theory and seeing real practice, our primary goal is to offer a textbook for advanced learners of the craft. Even now, as published authors with years of experience, the cases we acquired taught us a great deal.

From the position of teaching Creative Writing, rather than taking a purely academic position on *editing-as-craft*, this book aims to lay out some major notions and practices surrounding editing. Through cooperation with journal editors and individual writer-practitioners we have found quite singular and authentic practices, despite many common denominators, which show how the magic happens, how editors can transform a hot mess of words into a work of genius. Each chapter or case consists of the published text, a draft with visible edits and comments, a conversation with the editor and author about the process and specific issues that surfaced in the process, and in some cases even acquired email exchanges which highlight the unique author-editor relationship. The intention is that this will enable writers to see, in plain terms, what editing *looks like* – it can be complex, micro-focused, more concerned with nebulous concepts of authorial truth; it may be structural, or about internal cadence. Our aim is to demonstrate why the long road of rewriting is so important in our impatient twenty-first century, and to show students what they might train themselves to be alert to. In this volume, we want to pay as much attention to the relationships between authors and editors as we want to focus on the specific edits that bring to surface important issues of the art and craft of writing. To illustrate this, we'll look here at some interesting cases, both of successful and intimate relationships between authors and editors, and less encouraging ones.

We will now, in this introduction, say a few words about what we think editing is and why it is important. We'll begin with a metaphor. In her essay "The Blue of Distance," Rebecca Solnit writes:

> The strange resonant word *instar* describes the stage between two successive molts, for as it grows, a caterpillar . . . splits its skin again and again, each stage an instar. It remains a caterpillar as it goes through these molts, but no longer one in the same skin. There are rituals marking such splits, graduations, indoctrinations, ceremonies of change, though most changes proceed without such clear and encouraging recognition. *Instar* implies something both celestial and ingrown, something heavenly and disastrous, and perhaps change is commonly like that, a buried star, oscillating between near and far.
>
> *(Solnit 2006, 83)*

Instar, the terrifying process of destruction and creation in one, is an apt metaphor for the process of writing/rewriting – something of an aesthetic statement. But it is more than just the act of rewriting. Encouraging recognition of the process is important, the stages of transformation not accidental, the observation of them necessary, deserving, indeed demanding documentation, something that the editing process fixes. This is where we want to focus, not on nascent potential or finished beauty, but the process.

Observing *instar*, then. The constant oscillation between what we might consider the *near* of the writing experience and the more detached, more distant view of the editor, urging the splitting of skins. Or in rhetorical terms the paradigm between the form and the effect, both writer and ultimately editor turning *effect* into *affect*. At its most simplistic, we could say that editors deal in schemes (syntactic deviation), and writers deal in tropes (semantic deviation), although of course one is invariably changed by altering the other and so the process inevitably becomes a trading of affect and effect. Editing entails risks as well as benefits. Otherwise it would not be a form of art. It may often be a very precise undertaking, but one thing is certain, it cannot rely on mechanical thinking even when what seems to transpire looks like mechanics. There is no single formula that can, without problems, be applied to all texts. The more advanced the practitioner, the more intricate the process becomes.

Editing is an art, no doubt, but it is also a craft. And craft is something one learns with help from someone. Editors typically guide authors to insight about things such as content (e.g. too little or too much information, killing your darlings), language (how much one should be a slave to grammar, questions of authenticity and fresh-ness), flow (structure and pace of the text, cadences of sentences and paragraphs), style (consistency issues). The very notion of a *collaboration* between an author and an editor, whose goal is to perfect the manuscript in every way possible, was borne out of the technological changes coming from the late nineteenth century. What we commonly associate with the editing process – close attention to the text – was initially about spotting words that could cause public outcry. Barring partnerships and friendships between individuals, publishers would generally not get involved in the actual shaping of texts. There is very little information about those early pro-cesses, but what we do have mainly points to the specific things happening during the process of typesetting or conforming to particular in-house style. Jane Austen famously complained that two paragraphs were set as one and that a word was spelled differently (spelling was not standardized at the time), but she certainly did not have discussions on characterization or plot, which is a given in most modern editorial practice. In short, forms of *editing* that may have existed in early print culture remain something of a mystery.

The enormous influence that editors can have on both the work of single authors and fashionable styles is expressed by Louis Menand, who writes in *The New Yorker*:

> Writers are products of educational systems, but stories are products of mag-azine editorial practices and novels are products of publishing houses. Carver's minimalism was shaped by his editor, Gordon Lish, whom he met in Palo Alto in the nineteen-sixties. As an editor at *Esquire* and Knopf, Lish ... put a highly identifiable impress on American fiction, some of it by writers of lower-middle-class origin and some not. Robert Gottlieb, at Simon & Schuster, Knopf, and *The New Yorker*, surely had as much influence on the fiction that was written and published in the postwar period as anyone who taught at Iowa or Stanford.
>
> *(Menand 2009)*

Unsurprisingly, this influence is rarely straightforward. Success in one editorial partnership is not a guarantee of such in a second; Maxwell Perkins may have been a great editor of Hemingway, but arguably not as effective for Thomas Wolfe.

And what is the consequence of working *without* this difficult relationship, which ultimately can be seen to encourage "imaginative recklessness," to borrow Toni Morrison's phrase? We live in a time when everyone is published to an extent. The word "publish" is used in a much broader sense now, across different media, so one *publishes* both a Facebook post, a YouTube video, and a comment on social media. From Tweets and blogs to online zines, we leave traces of written materials everywhere. But equally, the services of professional editors are not an imperative part of this process. Two clicks and it is out there, your story, retweeted or cherrypicked or shared or liked, and all the other social media affirmations that have made anthimeric changes into actual acts of craft.

As teachers of creative writing, we have become increasingly aware that new technologies enable editing to become a more bare-faced practice. For example, Facebook's *editor* feature not only allows the person to change the text but also leaves a trail of changes so anyone can observe the process. In contrast, editing as a focused, taught, advanced-level skill features less than we would like within creative writing programmes. Where it is highlighted as part of the syllabus, it is more often than not relegated to a final, plenary session, a nod to the work that the student must pursue alone, drawn from some kind of writer's instinct. In the classroom, *process* is often talked about less than concrete narrative strategies: structure, voice, characterisation, perspective. It does not help that a good deal of online writing – professional newspapers and magazines excepted – is unedited. The immediate question for a writing tutor then, in the vein of the demise-of-editing prophecies, is: what is it that students are looking for from their finished work? Do we accept (or fail to notice) errors, typos, or syntactical clumsiness, because speed is so often of the essence, both in dissemination and in consumption? By and large, it used to be the case that short stories, the child of the new-print era magazine, *had* to pass through intensive scrutiny prior to publication. Twenty-first-century communication, on the other hand, encourages immediacy, and therefore perhaps facilitates a certain narrative imperfection. Paul Valery's notion that a work of art is never finished becomes truer than ever. The idea of an external eye, combing a story for flaws or flabbiness, becomes less a required or anticipated part of the process of taking the piece from final draft to publication (and in the majority of cases, we are aware this is what student writers are seeking). A new writer might publish several stories before encountering the more hands-on editing experience that was once standard.

To be fair, we are not arguing that online publishing leads to the dissemination of unpolished work. Both paying and non-paying markets take their work extremely seriously and a great deal of editing is involved in the production. In a podcast for *The Guardian* entitled "*The Art of Editing*", Alex Clark argues that the sheer size of conglomerate publishing, despite the means to invest, most resources go into (fewer) big works, with those lower on the "corporate ecology" not getting enough attention (11:19). He writes, "In more broad-brush terms the question is whether the image of the word-obsessed editor poring over a manuscript, red pen in hand, has given way to that of the whizz-bang entrepreneur attuned to the market's latest caprice, more at home with a tweet than a metaphor" (Clark 2011). If it is true that fewer stories are undergoing any kind of journal-side editing, and even fewer are really subjected to rigorous edits, one cannot but wonder what has been missed, or rather, where the editing takes place. The answer might often be in the classrooms of writing programmes, editorial services, and agents.

As editors, Durneen previously for *Short Fiction* in the UK, Mahmutović for *Two Thirds North* in Sweden, we are acutely aware that the well-known writer-reader relationships often tend to be the problematic ones. We have all read accounts by famous writers who speak of editors as those who destroy artistic integrity. 'Great art' is then produced in spite of these nemeses. As readers, however, we may side with Robert Gottlieb, who suggests in his Art of Fiction interview in *The Paris Review* that the editor's hand should be an invisible one (but nevertheless existent). And furthermore, as teachers, we are interested in the craft of editing, and specifically the diversity in the kind of role the editor might play in midwifing the text. The case studies we explore in this book demonstrate that it is not simply the relationship between author and editor that is so interesting, but the way individual texts themselves demand a different kind of intervention. It may be a structural element of the story that needs externally shoring up, or an issue with an ending. It might be a matter of voice, or a matter of what we might sweepingly call fictional truth.

Gottlieb, who has worked both as a book and magazine editor, takes this approach:

> Editing requires you to be always open, always responding. It is very important, for example, not to allow yourself to want the writer to write a certain kind of book. . . . You have to be inside *that* book and do your best to make it as good as it can be. And if you can't approach it in that spirit, you shouldn't be working on it. . . . No editor should work with a book he doesn't like, because his job as an editor is to make something better of what it is. If you try to turn a book into something it isn't, you're doomed to disaster.
>
> *(MacFarquhar 1994)*

One of our case studies from the journal *AGNI* shows a particularly close, working relationship between the editor Jennifer Drew and the writer Vince Passaro, deeply encouraging of Toni Morrison's notion of "reckless imagination." We have a unique access to Drew and Passaro's drafts and email exchanges, which enable us to follow the process in great detail and with transparency. Rather than simply identifying all the big and small changes, the difference between Draft A and Draft Z, here we could emphasise the *recognition* stage of Solnit's *instar* process that seems to be crucial for writers learning something about craft. Here both syntactic and semantic deviations are debated, the metamorphosis of the text active and organic and mutual. The dialogue shows not so much the changes made between drafts but the kind of discussion process involved regarding the final lines of Passaro's story:

> When I was younger, I thought it would cost me something, I thought it would drain me, diminish me, but I was wrong. Love is infinite and divisible,

and my greatest regrets are the moments I was not giving it sufficiently
to you.

The email dialogue goes as follows:

Passaro: Last line of the piece should be revised to read: "Love is infinite and divisible, and my greatest regrets TK TK the moments I was not giving it sufficiently
  to you." [sic] Here I need some advice. I don't like "are the moments" because
  it's weak and inaccurate: the regrets are not the moments. So "my greatest regrets
  arise from the moments"? abide in the moments? reside in the moments?
Drew: Love is infinite and divisible, and my greatest regrets are the moments I wasn't
  giving it sufficiently to you – is it too pedestrian to suggest Love is infinite and
  divisible, and my greatest regret is not giving it sufficiently to you? The moments
  add something, after the rest of that paragraph and its emphasis on moments, but
  maybe there again you don't need the moments after all? Though I also hate to
  lose regrets plural, if that is how one thinks of it. My greatest regrets are not
  giving it sufficiently?
Passaro: Actually how about this – just occurred to me – "Love is infinite and divisible,
  and what I regret most are the moments I was not giving it sufficiently to you."?
    No.
    "and my greatest regrets come from the moments I was not giving it suffi-
  ciently to you." either that or "arise from the moments." What do you think,
  between those two?

Abide in the moments. Reside in the moments. Arise from. The changes are small, but the
debate lengthy, involved, closely bound up with the text (Coleridge's infamous
"best words in the best order") examining rhythms and weightings (and in some
great detail later on, even the presence of certain commas) and something that perhaps cannot be easily quantified – emotional affect, the impact of the syntactical
change on the semantic effect. It is not lack of confidence on Passaro's part that he
asks for the advice, more the recognition of a need to sound it all out. Passaro refers
later to the different edits as the "Jen Variations," acknowledging both the imprint
she leaves on the finished story, and also how many possibilities exist before being
fixed in print form. Passaro understands the input at a different level.

  In creative writing classrooms, the question is whether new writers are actually equipped to ask the kind of questions that Passaro puts forward, to understand
that there is a "fundamental cohesion problem," even if unsure how to fix it.
Editing risks becoming an overly collaborative, pluralized act causing more confusion than effect. Student writers make changes because they are suggested by an
authority, not because they are necessary, and they do not always have (or sustain)
the confidence or the sensitivity to their own aesthetic to reject them even when
that would be appropriate. This seems to be at the heart of the craft and art of
editing, a fusion of scheme with trope where the two are themselves not visibly
divisible, always amplifying the thing the writer is trying to say, splitting away the

dead, stripping back the occlusion. Solnit's observation of *instar*, that same process of skin shedding, shape shifting, metamorphosis, form to effect, effect into affect, caterpillar to butterfly.

So how much should a new writer accept? For Gottlieb, adding any material would be an unacceptable intrusion. However, it depends, of course, if the addition is a requirement or a suggestion whose purpose is to indicate to the author how the editor is thinking in that particular case. The latter leaves the author with options, but does not show what type of addition the editor might accept. Here is an example of a story called "Ferðasaga" by Friðrik Sólnes Jónsson, which Mahmutović edited for *Two Thirds North 2013*. Jónsson's story was a fascinating, satirical look at tourism in Iceland. The editing involved much cutting but significantly, also two additions. We should note that Jónsson had worked on this story in one of Mahmutović's workshops but that it was only in the editing for publication that it transpired he had something of an aversion to making changes, partly due to the fact that Iceland did not have an active culture of editing, which left him unprepared for this process.

In order to understand why the following addition was suggested, some plot summary is in order. In this story, the tourist guide Mumjö joins Þorlákur, a bus driver, and a group of tourists, on a trip around Iceland. The story consists of a series of events largely filtered through Mumjö's peculiar mind. A major secondary character is a woman called "horseshoe woman," who sits right behind Mumjö and keeps pestering him with annoying questions. Then the story ends with a note. While abrupt endings are not a problem *per se*, this one seemed to be "unearned":

> Þorlákur came walking towards me. "Can you hear that?" I asked him. He stood for a while and listened with an expression of deep concentration on his face. I forced out a small but audible fart. He slapped my shoulder and giggled like crazy with squinted eyes. We climbed aboard the bus and waited for the tourists.
>
> Nothing else noteworthy happened on the trip and me and my dear flock of tourists parted ways as friends. But I try to remember only the good times. God knows that, and so does a single shy tear of joy that shivers with shame on a grateful cheek.

Mahmutović suggested deleting the final paragraph and wrote the suggestion below, with the following comment: "I added this because the question of the being-a-guide was always present and the woman played a big part in it, so in this way you can tie everything together a bit more. The added sentence is just a suggestion. Let me know if you have something else in mind." This proposed ending is in bold letters:

> Þorlákur came walking towards me. "Can you hear that?" I asked him. He stood for a while and listened with an expression of deep concentration on his face. I forced out a small but audible fart. He slapped my shoulder and giggled like crazy with squinted eyes. We climbed aboard the bus and waited for the tourists. **The horseshoe woman came to me and asked about**

the story behind xxx (NOTE: put something Icelandic here, something she'd be interested in).
"I don't know," I said. "Not everything in Iceland has a story."

The rewritten ending of the published story incorporates the suggestion in a way much better than the one the editor thought of:

The voice of the horseshoe woman sounded behind me, "That mountain is called Trölladyngja."

I yawned and asked her if anything interesting ever happened there. "I don't know," she said. "Not everything in Iceland has a story."

I smiled and signaled Þorlákur to start the engine. The din merged with the chatter of the tourists into white noise. In the distance, silver and gold stirred together with God's lovely light as the sun sank behind a cloud over a flat-topped mountain. My mindless body wobbled happily in its seat like pudding. The bodiless mind stared in front of the bus and the yellow lines in the middle of the road looked like the bus was flicking a thin yellow tongue. Then, I found myself standing at a decorated podium, wearing a pharaoh's headdress of gold and turquoise, and issuing some new decrees to throngs of people in a large square, encircled with colossal walls of stone. These good people, my flock, were going to finance the building of a sphinx with my face, larger than the one with the broken nose. The assemblage murmured discontentedly before joining together in a deafening uproar. I winked and snipers appeared on top of the surrounding walls and mowed down two thirds of the crowd. Silence. Then a low chant began among the survivors, growing louder and louder until they were all screaming at the top of their lungs in unison, and the chant went on escalating until my bus sailed into the next gravel parking lot in front of yet another rest stop. I muttered the chant clapping on my thighs to its rhythm as discreetly as I could so Þorlákur wouldn't notice: Mumjö! Mumjö! Mumjö! Mumjö! And I was thinking: *How did these worms enter me?*

(Jónsson 2013: 120)

Here we can see that the editor's note triggered something and the "horseshoe woman" did come back – but not to steal the ending. Rather we see Mumjö play along instead of the originally suggested brushing off, though the suggested sentence is kept almost verbatim. The extended paragraph reconnects the character to what he was thinking in the beginning of the story.

In comparison, let us look at a famous case of intrusive cutting: Carver vs. Lish. In her comparison of the edited and original texts of Carver's "So Much Water So Close to Home," Angela Readman writes: "When we talk about editing short stories, and we do, a lot, we talk about cutting every word that doesn't have to be in a story. But I'm not sure it's always so simple." Mostly, we assume, it is the question of shooting adverbs and killing darlings, and in some cases, such as Carver, enormous deletions of content. The question of what is gained and what is lost is most important. Readman discusses the following original passage from "So Much Water So Close to Home":

> I close my eyes for a minute and hold onto the drainboard. I must not dwell on this any longer. I must get over it, put it out sight, out of mind, etc and "go on". I open my eyes. Despite everything, knowing all that may be in store, I rake my arm across the drainboard and send dishes and glasses smashing and scattering across the floor.
>
> He doesn't move ... I hate him for that, not moving ... The wind takes the smoke out of his mouth in a stream. Why do I notice that? He can never know how much I pity him for that, for sitting still and listening, and letting the smoke stream out of his mouth.

The published version reads as follows:

> I close my eyes and hold onto the sink. Then I rake my arm across the drainboard and send the dishes to the floor. He doesn't move. I know he's heard.
>
> *(Readman 2014)*

For Readman, the action is the same, but the loss is great because we lose the female perspective, which would add complexity and depth to the narrative. The male character, in the other edits, is more conflicted. Overall, "the longer story is both more brutal *and* more tender" (Readman 2014). While the story is strong in its edited version, there is no doubt that the cuts alter the characters and the story as such. The content may seem the same but it is not. The story has a different sensibility. It shows a different type of masculinity and femininity from Carver's original intention.

Since much editing is a reaction to overwriting, the question of excess is omnipresent within various MFA programmes and among most professionals. Less is more seems to be the guiding principle for a great deal of modern writers and editors. The question is, how do we teach beginners to edit their own work following this principle, but without pushing them over into editing their stories to death. Sometimes, as you will see in the fourth case in this volume, "King of the Ball," a cut that fixes the flow may disrupt the authenticity and the solution is far more complex, demanding a true collaboration rather than just 'accept-deny'. No doubt, many published stories *feel* like they could be trimmed some. This is not necessarily a minimalist idea. But what might be seen as overwriting for Lish, is over-editing for Readman.

The questioning of cutting, adding, and being too intrusive seems to suggest something we might call the *ethics of editing*. Can we reach a consensus on any threshold in the editing process beyond what individual authors and editors find acceptable? It would be hard, given that there is little public discourse on how much is "too much," and it would be hard to quantify it anyway. Most successful cases we have garnered for our book show there is either an existing relationship between an editor and an author, or a particular relationship that grows through the process of writing, rewriting, and editing, which is something few can afford or have the opportunity to invest in. From the given examples, we have seen that different practitioners have different routines and values. We assume then that there is no such thing as 'too little' if the editor does not find it necessary to suggest anything. In fact, as mentioned earlier, many journals are looking for stories that need neither editing nor proofreading. The real question we need to ask is: when does an editor stop being an editor and become the writer of the story?

The truth is, this may be hard to determine, unless we accept it as one of those *I know it when I see it* type of judgments. We assume most of us would recoil at wholly rewriting a text, or changing the style, and yet the types of edits performed by Lish on Carver and Pound on Eliot, even when only concerned with cuts, do not simply help shape the text but also both the content and the style. Eliot dedicated *The Waste Land* to Pound as "a better craftsman." Was Lish a better craftsman than Carver? Much of what we now 'recognise' as Carver is largely due to Lish's interventions. As Readman shows, this is not only the question of style but also characterisation and plotting, because all the elements of craft that go into a work of art, especially in dense, short fiction with a lot of subtext, are so tightly connected that one cannot really pull one string without changing (although not necessarily ruining) the tapestry.

In our own practice, minding the style of the author has always been a hard limit. If the edit changes the style into something else then we are already speaking about rewriting, which, as an editorial practice, seems extreme. And yet, is not a change of a single word already a form of rewriting? Does not an accepted suggestion from an editor already constitute co-writing, an act of translation from one conceived version to another perceived one? Or can this be likened more readily to the relationship between musician and producer, a sharpening of the link between technique and affect, a way of making visible the invisible, the same act of amplification we were able to see in the working relationship between Drew and Passaro? Understood this way, it is clear we need to be speaking of scales of involvement, from few word changes to practical ghostwriting. Gottlieb says,

> When I worked with Margaret Atwood at *The New Yorker*, for instance, whether there was a plot problem or a punctuation problem, if the solution came from her it worked wonderfully. But if I offered one myself, it never took. . . . Your job as an editor is to figure out what the book needs, but the writer has to provide it.
>
> *(MacFarquhar 1994)*

At what level on a scale from minimum to maximum lies Carver's collaboration with Lish? Eliot's work with Pound? The grounding notion of an editor as an invisible hand, whether in a journal or a publishing house, or within the commercial structures of modern writers' services, seems to be permanently valid, accepted,

unquestioned. For this reason, the fact that the contributors to our project on editing have opted to offer their knowledge and their archives to anyone who seeks to
improve as a writer, editor, or both, is truly admirable. What is needed is more
transparency that shows possibilities for learning, potential traps, gains and losses.
There are no formulae and mathematical precision after all.

References

Clark, Alex (2011), "The Lost Art of Editing," *The Guardian*. Online at www.theguardian.
com/books/2011/feb/11/lost-art-editing-books-publishing. Accessed 9 June 2015.

Jónsson, Friðrik Sólnes (2013), "Ferðasaga," *Two Thirds North*, pp. 103–121.

MacFarquhar, Larissa (1994), "Robert Gottlieb, The Art of Editing No. 1," *The Paris Review*,
Spring. Online at www.theparisreview.org/interviews/1760/the-art-of-editing-no-
1-robert-gottlieb. Accessed 15 May 2015.

Menand, Louis (2009), Online at www.newyorker.com/magazine/2009/06/08/show-or-
tell.

Morrison, Blake (2005), "Black day for the Blue Pencil," *The Observer*, August. Online at
www.theguardian.com/books/2005/aug/06/featuresreviews.guardianreview1. Accessed
8 June 2015.

Readman, Angela (2014), "What We Talk About When We Talk About Editing," *Thresholds
Forum*. Online at http://blogs.chi.ac.uk/shortstoryforum/what-we-talk-about-when-
we-talk-about-editing/. Accessed 20 December 2014.

Solnit, Rebecca (2006), "The Blue of Distance," *A Field Guide to Getting Lost*. London:
Canongate, pp. 65–83.

2

"FINAL INSTRUCTIONS FOR MY DISPOSAL"

AGNI Magazine

Vince Passaro and Jennifer Alise Drew

This case is as interesting for the debate it sparks regarding authorial intention as it is for the line-by-line edits themselves. It is a story that veers towards memoir and Drew never loses sight of that fact. She is mindful of the impact of certain fictional revelations in the narrative and concerned that the urge to confess, manifested by Passaro's narrator, might not be fully in the best interests of either the narrative integrity or that of its author. In tracing the conversations surrounding the refinement of the piece from the point it lands in Drew's inbox, we see real concern for shaping the story into something that maintains its original purpose while softening its raw edges. Sometimes these changes are more significant, the removal of certain details to defuse a scene, for example. In other places, they operate at micro level. One sentence is debated over several days, in order to land on the precise word order required to strike the right note home.

The role of editor in this case study may be viewed as somewhat protective, seeing things that the writer simply could not, and making them visible, or invisible as the case may be. The final revisions ultimately come from Passaro himself, Drew's job here being more to ask new drafts to step into the room of their own accord rather than insist they look a particular way. But the wider email dialogue surrounding the edits raises a different question too, and one of whether or not the editor equally has what we might see as a duty to "hold the line" and establishes the value and power of the non-mechanical aspects of editing. Last minute changes on the part of the writer are described at one stage in the email exchange as "retreats" and "the children of cold-feet re-readings." Here is where we see the editor intervene and resist the same temptation to tweak, re-tweak and adjust for which Alice Munro was infamous. There is an implication, worthy of further debate, that only from without, from the dispassionate perspective of the scheme as a whole, can such cold-feet errors be avoided.

This case study shows us, amongst other things, that editing is not simply about pulling apart, or letting things emerge, but preserving what is there. "Your edits are outstanding," says Passaro to Drew, "in recognizing, in a way I could never quite figure out, some fundamental cohesion problem in the stance of the piece." Passaro's words seem crucial. *In a way I could never quite figure out.* Here is the nub of it. Drew's eye is key to delivering the story successfully. It is a gaze that is full of intent, yet detached, nudging Passaro to ask the right questions of himself something that can be hard to have confidence in as a student writer rather than imposing them directly. In this case, the cohesion extends to the relationship between editor and writer, not just the narrative itself, and reminds us why this previously routine aspect of the path to publication remains so important even when the option to bypass it exists.

"Final Instructions for My Disposal"

To my children, to N, to a few other people who shall for now remain nameless – maybe later I'll be able to name you, but currently it requires more in the way of moral resources than I have on hand.

Hear ye.

We exist physically at the molecular level; we are comprehensible as strings of protein; so, when it comes to my "remains" as they are called, for Christ's sake, just get on with it, send me to the fires. I'm fifty-four now, with gray hair and gray beard, neatly trimmed for the most youthful effect a gray beard can have, and, to further express my youthful self-state – every middle-aged man's accessory if he can't afford a European sports car – a young child, the newest of you, a highly enjoyable three-year-old boy who still speaks of me in generally positive terms. It occurred to me that I should write a little testament and make known to all of you my wishes regarding the usual: the tubes in and hoses out, the interment, and the division of my meager collection of stuff, my items, the things that might be of interest or stir desire. Cash I assume there'll be none of – you know me – but I'll mention it later just in case.

~

First: put my ashes in a silver Illy can. I prefer the espresso grind with the black stripe. You can bury it in the yard, if we ever manage to have a yard. Or, take it out to sea. I don't think I ever shared with you my distant and lazy fondness for the sea. I read a lot of Conrad, not to mention Melville. Do you know about *Hornblower*? And *Mutiny on the Bounty*? (All three volumes.) *Two Years Before the Mast*? I bet not. The YA novels of American pirates running the British blockades off the coast of New England in 1812 – I never forced any of this upon you, not as I did Twain and *The Call of the Wild*. I still love boats, still wish I could sail. All a surprise to you.

But maybe you'd like to do something more literary. Hire some grad student to spread the ashes discreetly around Flannery O'Connor's farm in Milledgeville, which is open to the public now. I am what I am, or was what I was, to the extent I ever managed to be it, because of her.

Or – here's what I'd like best, actually. Take the Illy can to "1020," the tavern at that address on Amsterdam Avenue at the corner of 110th Street – you know the place, I believe one or two of you have begun to frequent it since I left the neighborhood – and put what's left of me on the bar in the front corner where the painter, George the Czech, usually sits (he'll approve – if he's not in Ecuador where he spends half the year with his twenty-five-year-old mestiza girlfriend and new baby, about whom his divorced wife and teenage children in New York, last I heard, knew not a thing). Take me there and set me up with a Jameson straight up, a cold lager, a notebook, a Waterman, a 2B drawing pencil, a pack of Lucky Strikes, and a Leica CL. Use your iPhones to take pictures of this tableau. Send the images to all my friends.

> Memories of booze and expanded time and tea-gold light forcing itself through the street-side windows of the bars I've known on empty afternoons. No more alcohol for me, you know. Oh what a story that is. Except it isn't. It's just an unpleasant, mildly pathetic sequence of events, the kind that passes through your mind when you're stepping over a dirty raincoat abandoned on the sidewalk. Whatever the story is, you don't actually want to know it.

The main point: once you have the ashes, whichever of you takes them from the dyshidrotic hands of the funeral director, probably not old, probably surprisingly young, the business has to have some young people in it after all, do not leave them sitting around and you feeling all guilty because you haven't done something suitable with them. If you leave them sitting around then just do that. Move them from one closet to another every decade or so until you die. The main thing is, don't feel guilty. Move on. Memory will speak what it speaks. Memory is the eternity we sometimes wish for. It has enormous vacancies in it, just like the universe – these are the collapsed black gravitational centers of longing. Memory is malleable, as would be any narrative taking place outside time; it, or parts of it, can happen over and over, and, even with different outcomes, all the contingencies will remain intact – I wish I'd been able to see this earlier. Even now, I wish I could keep it in my head. Uncountable alternate universes full of the choices that, in this universe, no one made. But this is just the kind of hey-the-present-lasts-forever momentary revelation you cannot, by virtue of being human, keep in your head. Because, hello, here is life: you still have to sit on hold with the fucking insurance company. You still have to go to CVS and face Drugstore World, where language seems no longer to function as elsewhere, where no one ever understands what the fuck you're asking for. The products they sell? Never heard of them. Customers? Never heard of them. You still – in other words – have to deal with the daily matrix of enslaving bureaucracies, the enormous exhausting relentless forces aimed, with no admitted authorship, at dehumanizing you and destroying life's possibilities for meaning. All wisdom vanishes. That's the point. *If* you could touch the immanent God in every aspect of the universe, *if* you could see God and talk to God – and that is what an infinite awareness would entail – would you ever say, hold on, I have to do my taxes? Wait, I have to deal with these fucking e-mails, let me get back to you this afternoon? Would you go to work? Would you come home? No. Wrapped in nothing but the divine, you would howl on the sidewalks and grab people wild-eyed, you would be picked up and taken to Bellevue, you would starve, your teeth would fall out – you would die. God is the sun, life is the glass: you're the ant.

If none of the above works for you, just spread me out around one of the elms in Riverside Park, north of 105th and south of 116th, if you can manage it, or down on the softball fields near there, by the highway and the river, where Richard Hart and Tom Adams (two properly disheveled sons of New Orleans) and I used to play every Thursday and Friday over the summer of 1980, after late breakfast at The Mill Luncheonette, because none of us had all that much to do – there was a paralyzing recession on, but life was cheap and I remember these days as long hours of freedom, in fact I remember specifically enjoying them as such, noting the freedom, tasting it as if it were a grandmother's famous sauce, as if I already knew its time had run out. Occasionally in those pick-up games I hit the ball off the high wall in left, sometimes halfway up; only twice did I see anyone hit it over, up onto the promenade – anyway, if I'm there, and you ever feel the need to visit, you'll know where to go. Be done with it in any case. I won't care. By then I'll be wherever it is I'm supposed to be. If you can, pray for me. I have for you.

~

But I've gotten ahead of myself. When I'm going out – the awful part, the part with various terrifying and disgusting smells and the need for professionals just to clean up – revive me if it's worthwhile, don't if it's not. I'm sorry I can't be more specific, but that's all I can say about it really. If you make the wrong decision, don't worry, it's not a big deal, because here's one sure fact: I'm going to die at some point. I'd prefer to go by reason of forces other than the *fill-out-the-forms-and-sign-here* version of bureaucratized volition. (Nietzsche identified the birth of tragedy but who at any length has remarked its death, its utter exclusion, its impossibility?) If I'm in a nice coma and don't need breathing equipment, etc., just a discreet feeding tube, then leave me there, because who knows what that's all about. I might be finding something out. You never know. Caverns of silence. Charcoal darkness. Phosphorescent fish with shallow cavities where their ancestors' eyes would have been. Skip the big efforts, let me lie there, no one can bother me anymore. A quick twice-weekly phone chat with the nurses will do. Or email. Friend them on Facebook. You don't have to visit. If you're worried about the solitude, hour upon hour upon hour of it, don't. I never worry about solitude. If you're still worried, tell the nurses to use my room to smoke cigarettes or dip snuff or drink vodka or whatever other illicit shit they might like to do, perhaps they need just a simple place to gather and complain about the others. To play rummy. To fondle (or worse) their colleagues. Tell them I smile upon them. Tell them I'm happy for them. I'll enjoy the conversation. All those accents. They'll all be saying to each other forget it all the time. "Forget it girl, it won't never be no different," and that last will have all three of its God-given syllables . . . *Won't never be no diff-er-ahnt*. If you do visit – please sing. You all have such beautiful voices.

> *The boy – fifth grade, or sixth, twelve years old, stands before the choir in the apse of the great cathedral, on which low central ground, but for the highest masses, the weekly altar is laid. He sings a Magnificat, "My soul . . . doth magnify the Lord," in a voice pure and powerful. A high G of piercing beauty. He does not want to be there. His life is a series of oppressions: home, school, choir. He has perfect pitch. His talents, his skills, his various forms of brilliance daily conspire to punish him. He has a flawless calm before the crowd. He sings, perfectly, as once, much younger, eight or nine, he had played a Bach piece for violin, at just that fine cusp of perfection that can still a room. After: no elation. This is what is required? This is what the music requires, what the audience requires, what you expect? Okay. Here.*

Death, unconsciousness, stands as relief from the harrowing memories of failure, of humiliation, of almost incomprehensible mistakenness: think of it, these things will be lifted from me, and someday too from you, as when the beautiful hostess takes your coat at a restaurant and smiles.

My funeral arrangements: now, about this, I have to say I'm feeling somewhat particular. Invite all the women. I'm serious. I want them all beckoned – some of them will come – going back to college days. Or, no: grade school. I want a large venue, many speakers; I want you strongly to encourage the comic, the inappropriate, the nakedly sentimental. Invite the hostile: *You know, I have to say, he annoyed the shit out of me.* There are some people who really hate me. Invite them to speak. Certain mystifyingly successful writers of sodden forgettable sentences. Let them have at me. That'll wake people up. *What a lazy, deluded, superior, pompous fucktard. I hated the fucking guy. Glib and lazy. What did he ever do? I won the Pulitzer Prize for Christ's sake, what did he win?* I want lots of music. I want everyone to sit there and listen to all thirty-two minutes of "Mountain Jam," from the Allman Brothers at Fillmore East. Tell people to bring drugs. Make it a party. Everyone should take some Ecstasy. X. In our day it had four letters – MDMA, something like that. Then it was a drug, now it's a combined degree. Anyway, shock people: make the papers, pass some joints around. Open bar in the rear two corners . . . I suppose such things cannot happen anymore. Well, someone, before the day is over, at least one poor schmuck whom everyone will later ridicule, should drunkenly insist on a return to freedom. Just for the hell of it.

~

So: I brought up the women. There are things I want you to know, but not really. I want you to glimpse the silhouette of a few things, that's all. What do any of us want to say in the end? I lived. I walked the planet. I made a few amusing remarks. I was loved. For a while after, I was remembered.

And let it be known: I loved them all. Andrea (who by her friends was called, without irony, Cookie), and Anna, and Ruth, and Gabrielle, and Laura, and Laureen and also a Lorene which makes no sense but she was from Dallas; Maureen Noreen Cynthia Deirdre Cathy Katherine Annaliese Karen Susan. Two Susans, actually. The first was a student of mine, the only student I ever fell for; I was only thirty – a forgivable age for that particular sin. There was a Jenn, with two *n*'s, who knows why. I never asked. Alex, Alison, Oleh. Two Amandas and two Joannas. And two Victorias, both dark-eyed, soft-skinned, proud, ambitious girls.

> *Tonight I'm at the counter, peeling fava beans, thinking of Debra Kelly. First love. Third grade. I was almost sick to my stomach every day. I was ill with it, literally. She ended up studying in Maine and becoming a dancer, which makes sense, one thinks of the way she stood there: her shoulders straight and her yellow hair clipped on each side and fanned across her back, which curved inward toward the base of the spine, not a sway-backed curve just a subtle perfect line; and the plaid Catholic school skirt centered and holding there on her hips though she was always thin, and then – but what? We were eight years old? Nine? I couldn't take my eyes from her, except I couldn't keep them on her either, I felt as if I'd start to dissolve like a lump of powdered soap under a faucet. Her skin was pale and softly defined and utterly unblemished. I decided to write a long note to our teacher, a large woman with a stiff short hairdo the color of gold spray paint, an imposing bosom that stuck out like a shelf, and much, much perfume. Generally stern, she was most kind to me on several fraught occasions, and shocked me once with an iron hug from the desk after calling me up to the front and announcing some score I'd gotten on a standardized test. I asked my mother what it was like, to be in love, and she started quizzing me with altogether too much amusement, so, having no one else, I took it to Mrs. Bross – asking to be transferred to the other third grade class because I just couldn't concentrate. . . . This had been going on for at least four or five days. Maybe more. Maybe close to two weeks! Such a sweet, slow annihilation. I could not believe how good this form of torment felt, how utterly addictive. But then – wisdom – I decided to ride it out and not give Mrs. Bross that note, which would have been one of those childhood social missteps, a knife in the memory that one regrets right into the grave. I have enough of those already. But this Debra Kelly and I were in a crowd later, in high school, or, rather, she occasionally deigned to join our crowd for a movie or a party, and talking to her remained a matter of taking my palpitating venous sense of identity into my hands and squishing it. (You can imagine the sound.) She was the only tall blonde woman I ever loved.*
>
> *The next year came Maureen Pappianous. Gleaming black hair. While playing one day in the basement of her apartment building, she was burned badly by a hot water pipe breaking; she was a dark sparkling girl, shy, and kind, ever after with scarred skin along her right side, over her lower neck and shoulder and arm and probably parts of her side and back and who knows where else. She was intensely beautiful, half Irish, half Greek; tonight, thinking of her, it all dovetails nicely, the ten-year-old's built-in*

knowledge of enormous shapeless impossibility, and the later version, the midlife, hard-bordered, supremely familiar sense of impossibility: time don't go that way, brother. The sense of nostalgia and loss — all this makes a fine piece of furniture for the spirit. At such moments one knows one is alive. I sat behind her (blessed alphabet); I liked to touch her hair, ever so lightly, touching a part of her but she couldn't feel it. I did accents of the world. She and the girl beside me — whom I can't remember at all, name, face, nothing — loved this; they would request countries and I would do them. All imitations from the 4:30 movies. They could have flummoxed me so easily, what did I know of the world? They could have said Hungary or Tibet or Thailand, but of course they were no more sophisticated than I was — it was fourth grade after all — nor, it occurs to me, did they want me to fail. We men, we want each other to fail, it's wired in, you fail, I might succeed, or I will look less bad failing. But the girls don't want us to fail. This is something that men don't realize, especially after all the cruelties and rejections of adolescence: women would prefer we succeed and will help us to do so, as long as we don't catch them at it.

Of course, yes, I know, there are always exceptions.

To my ex-wife I leave a list of ragged questions: Why did we do that to each other? And to our children? Did we believe that we and they would just somehow survive all that violence? I remember only the color red. The rage and blood, you with something sharp, anything that came to hand, and your wild, murderous eyes. Please give your answers to my attorney. He will lock them in a file for fifty years and then they will be destroyed.

So you know I grew up alone with two women. Two Irish women, who revealed little of the truth about themselves. I suspect this partly accounts for the way I've been driven to study women my whole life, read them as though they were difficult books. I am captured by them still — I'm old, but it turns out I'm not over the worst of it — I love to watch the way they move, certain gestures, how they twist around to see the backs of their legs. When you live with a woman — N, this is true of you — you learn that she holds herself differently depending on what she's wearing. It's a rare woman who looks right standing naked putting a kettle on for tea. In skirts, with heels, your body, not just your appearance but seemingly your actual *self*, is different from how you are in pajama pants and a borrowed shirt. In your feet, that's where you cannot hide: you, every woman, your feet express you in a kind of footy semaphore, minute by minute, small boned, fine muscled, elaborate. And there's more, of course: the way you tilt your heads back slightly to put on makeup; the way you put a hand up — not all do this, but many — while you're chewing, even if you're not talking or laughing and your lips are closed. N, you do it when you speak at the table. My mother (aha! you all say; well, fuck you, aha yourself) sitting with her legs crossed, putting on lipstick or smoking a cigarette or sipping cold whiskey that looked brown and clear as a mountain stream — the ice made a sound like money in the glass. Her hands, small and slender and white. She smoked filterless Raleigh cigarettes and would from time to time pick a bit of tobacco from her lips or from the tip of her tongue, a gesture redolent of adulthood and sexuality. Ah, they fuck you up. It got a lot worse than that, too — I mean that kind of thing is child's play compared to what came later. There are things I haven't told you, boys, and likely won't — you would not feel enlightened by it, and, really, the details don't matter: it was a complex, impacted, damaging relationship; I had a simpler but just as damaging relationship with my old man. Of course being grown-up entails the long struggle to decide to try to get over it. But first we must reenact it, over and over, repeat the mistake until we know it, until we can see the thing: the outline of the dragon.

> He stands in the kitchen in the evening, listening to her put their boy to bed; he is rinsing a plate in soft running water and there washes over him a sense of the extraordinary privilege of the moment, her love of their child, the ease of their gracious apartment and their KitchenAid dishwasher which they use every day, after eating their fill, every day. Behind this thought crouches an abiding fear: that it is, all of it, undeserved, that it is unfair, that it will be taken away.

Him: that's me. But it's also not. This scene never happened. We don't have a KitchenAid dishwasher, that's just invention; we detest the cheap dishwasher we do in fact have, which came with the place and which, N will verify, is growing some sort of intractable mold around the base of the inner chamber. I'm often at the sink while she is putting our boy to bed but this particular moment of fear, notwithstanding all the moments of fear one endures through the day, this one did not happen. Yet it did happen, to me, in the fact of writing it; because to write something in fictional mode that is at least minimally convincing, paradoxically requires that one experience it, whereas this is, again paradoxically, *not* required when one writes convincingly in memoir: the simple announcement at the outset that *all this really happened* lifts the obligation of flawless accuracy. One must only master the voice of memory: *In the evenings I stood at the sink and listened to her put our boy to bed, she knew his books by heart, quoted them to him while she washed him and picked up his toys.* One does not have to experience or re-experience that moment. In that sentence, in fact, the rituals are out of order, one could not be experiencing it while writing it; but to the reader it is convincing enough, memory is enough: the past has proved itself; the present, contingent, like fiction, has not.

And this, the creation of the real, which is not real but must be real — it's an interesting way to live. Alas, just as with talking to God, it does keep you from your responsibilities. Even now, at this late date, I want you to know me. This is overbearing, I realize.

~

So, what is at the core of life but love? An image I cannot shake: a man, my age, kissing a woman in Grand Central. She was a beautiful woman. I think of it now every time I'm there, in that part of the station.

She was waiting for him when he came off the train; she'd arrived a day or two before from upstate, where she'd been staying, but he couldn't get away until the Thursday; so they met that day in the famed terminal, at the last ticket booth, which is always closed – most of them are closed now – a curiously private nook of tinted marble and cast-iron window grates in a vast and definitively public space. They stood and stared, searching; a look of pleasure. Eyes alight. Sadness and pleasure. This thing they had, this affair of letters and a few illicit phone calls, was doomed, they'd agreed it was doomed, but here they were at another moment in which loss is built into the fervent anticipation. They kissed. He couldn't believe her mouth. It had been twenty-five years since they'd met, been introduced – by whom? – and they'd spoken then only briefly, graduate students at the university, standing in the ratty coffee lounge, a room in which he could not remember ever having been unhappy. He was second-year, slightly older than most, twenty-nine, outwardly confident, accomplished; she was young, the youngest person there, a prodigy. Hers was the kind of beauty that is connected to – is inseparable from – an immutable core, a self; her face was a little crooked and animated by a light you were bathed in the minute you engaged with her or saw her smile. She was immediately striking. She had that hair. She had those sad vivid mischievous eyes. She was not that tall and neither thin nor heavy; she was solid, rounded, sturdy, voluptuous. She was not one whose fire needed to be lit; it was burning already. They might have seen each other once or twice again after that, but neither remembered anything except the first meeting, brief, compelling. She told him that she'd seen him and thought, I'd like to sleep with him.

They went to lunch and then to a hotel, expensive and thoroughly adequate. They kept having to heave aside the pillows, which were the size of Labradors and seemed forever to be getting in the way: except then suddenly she'd grab one, with urgency and impassioned expertise, and jam it beneath her in just the right way to ease some conundrum they were working through. He watched her desire, studied it; he had trouble believing in it, but there it was, undeniable. She was in an open marriage. Mainly she dated younger men: they had, she'd said archly, a certain vigor. This irritated him, of course. His irritation made her glad and he knew it would make her glad so it made him glad too. Later he was above her and she began using her muscles to grip him – hard, really hard – and he looked at her and said I didn't know you knew how to do that, and she laughed and said well I'm glad you can feel it, the twenty-eight-year-olds never seem to notice. . . . He had never felt so at ease with someone new: all his life. Of course, he would realize much later, the person he was finally at ease with was himself. They used condoms. Even this didn't bother him though normally it would. He couldn't come but he didn't mind because it meant they could fuck more. After every respite a new condom. It was comical and vulgar, the wrappers dropped around the big bed. A week or two after she'd returned home, she wrote him that she was dropping her kids somewhere, to hip-hop dance class or aikido or lacrosse; she said they parked, and before anyone was out of the car in this flash moment came a sharp memory of being in bed with him, and she made an involuntary sound, like ooph – but they didn't hear her. They are both boys, he wanted to say, they will never hear you in that way, but she wouldn't believe that. A girl would have heard it instantly, would have known there was something in it. But not the boys. Off they went. . . . She'd told him in bed on the second day that she wanted him to fuck her in the ass and he did and here, this, now, finally he was able to come, his broad peasant hand holding the headboard slamming into her. Of course there was lubricant so he left his handprint on the fabric of the headboard, which was not really a headboard but an attractive cloth-covered board attached to the wall behind the bed. Now it was like the caves in France: he had left evidence of his existence there. When she pointed it out to him he suggested he draw a deer and a figure shooting it with an arrow.

And so once again in life he found it necessary to acknowledge a broader definition of love. He loved her; they loved each other; it was insane, after just a couple of months of correspondence and these two days in New York, it wasn't the way they loved other people but it stood between them, undeniable, this shocking, heated intimacy in a shared language.

Then one day, for her, it was over. Whatever this was they'd been feeling, she couldn't feel it anymore. He stopped hearing from her. He was stunned at first: no one had ever dumped him before, not unless he'd arranged it. In the first weeks he could hardly stand it: existence. It was awful. It made him sick and then put him in pain and he felt as though every nerve ending along the surface of his skin was mildly burning: he hurt, his whole person hurt. For there was something altered in him in the wake of this intense, passing moment, despite its brevity and unreality; something that was corporal, central, undeniable – no matter the pitfalls we have to call it his heart (yes, it's a cliché, yes, his heart) – a muscle at the core of him that pushed his blood around and helped him breathe and allowed him to love and laugh and fuck and rarely, once a decade, weep – and a fresh little piece of it was broken off now, spalled, chipped, dead on the floor, lying there, and under this new light he could see not just those fragments but the poor old organ itself: it was cracked in other places and worn; and plainly its new injuries marked one more step in life, one more chunk of time, which kept moving, tumbling, rolling, skidding, toward some inevitable finish, a completion, an ending – which he could not imagine, but which he now believed, when it finally came, he would not fear.

There it is: don't grow old with an unblemished heart. Be free. Don't be afraid of dying.

~

We have not yet spoken of the books or the cameras or the lenses or the nice art supplies and Waterman pens or the four-and-a-half feet of old journals. Just decide among yourselves. Anything someone wants he should have. If more than one want it, add it to a pile to be considered later; trade and barter one thing against another. Divide among you equally my reputation, such as it is, and use it as sunscreen. The language, the images, the rights, the proper disposition: I can see that it will be remarkable to me and others how little interest my work will have for me when I'm dying. I shall assign a literary executor: to this person please deliver the journals, and don't think about them anymore. If something of them gets published, don't worry about it. After two weeks it's forgotten and really, even from the first, no one gives a shit. Secrets are a dream.

Of course, there's no money, that's the upshot. You certainly won't be surprised. I have a nice insurance policy at work, a hefty sum if there were only one of you, but divided four ways it is more like part of a down payment on a house. In a previous decade. Anyway, there's that. Try to be happy.

(Okay, here: if you're interested in money, each of you is quite sufficiently smart to make plenty of it. Only self-consciousness and perhaps aesthetic and moral and cultural distaste, as well as raw fear, fear of raising your middle finger to God and humanity, stand in the way of amassing large sums of money. But if money is what you want, all these impediments, moral, aesthetic, blah blah, can be jettisoned.

I don't remember ever meeting anyone who'd made large sums of money, on purpose, who was also imaginative. Just imitate. That's what they all do.)

In the end, it would be a boon if we were able to enjoy our own existence, as those who've loved us have enjoyed us. Let me try to give you that, since as of now, it's clear, I have little else to give you. Let me tell you that I love you; and that I admire you. That you have sharp minds, sharp tongues, and, best of all, sharp consciences. You love the woods. You can make music. You understand complex numbers and simple machines. You are kind to children. You believe there is beauty in the world, and you pursue it.

~

Well boys let me disclose the gifts reserved for age. First, self-forgiveness comes on slowly but pointedly, like a brief, recurring memory of childhood happiness. It's nice. Second, the treasures of solitude are best enjoyed in youth; I have come to recognize that my drive for solitude, in middle life and beyond, is a poisonous addiction. Third, and related to the second, to seek others and then to push them away is, first of all, mean and unfair; but for you, if you're the one doing it, it's like rowing one way with the left arm, the other way with the right. Having gotten nowhere and gained nothing, you're still exhausted.

I realized something last year when I served as best man at the wedding of my friend T. He came, as did I, from an unstable and ultimately shattered set of circumstances. Nevertheless he has made himself into a funny, generous, kind, and only mildly neurotic adult. His wedding took place downtown, one block from the site of the World Trade Center. Over the days before the wedding, as I compressed various thoughts, aiming toward some vague preparedness to make a toast, it came to me that in recent years I've gotten to know some young people, decent, smart, talented, likeable, from stable and prosperous homes, and in knowing them I became aware of the basic position of security upon which they stood to face the world: you, my older sons, mostly don't have it, I never had it, and T, if possible, had it even less; people such as he and I were dropped into our adulthoods and had to face the dilemma of building strong and secure identities – in relation to the world, its indifference, our desires – with nothing at all supporting us; whereas some other people have solid ground beneath them. It's a commonplace notion, I'd just never really taken it in before. And the image that followed was that of Philippe Petit, who crossed between the towers on a high wire the year I came to New York (I was eighteen, recently orphaned, completely set loose in the world). The images of Petit on the wire remained vivid for me all these years, a prominent part of my inner iconography, and suddenly I understood, at least in part, why: this was us, I told T in the toast, hanging between those absurd and beautiful towers; Petit represented people like us, achieving our existence, our sense of who we are, when he was dancing out there in gray light with nothing but a hundred stories of air beneath him, facing a forty-mile-an-hour wind.

Flannery O'Connor several times in her letters quoted the French (very Catholic) writer François Mauriac's advice for the artist: "Purify the source." That's a lifetime's project. The first requirement is surviving your high-wire walk to selfhood. And then, one strategy might be (I certainly haven't gotten there and can't say for sure) to look toward what you want. Move toward what you want. But while you're doing that, work on wanting the right things. Never relent. After you give up, go back. Give up again, go back again. I am often slowed to a crawl by a sense that what I want to do is too hard; I'm too soft; it's not worth it; it's futile. Then I go back.

Once we're older – very few people from middle age onward won't claim this – youth and its problems seem to scream out for our advice. It all looks so clear to us now, so much more manageable than it is when you're in it. But the advice we have to offer is almost entirely ridiculous. It's like telling a drowning man all he needs to do is swim.

Nevertheless here I go.

When people tell you they love you: listen to them.

Don't dismiss it, or think them foolish. Try to see yourself as they see you. Just for a moment. Realize the dignity you have, struggling in the world, most days with some tangible grace. Realize your courage. See the beauty, your own beauty. Do this just for a moment – you only need a moment. But do it over and over, and over and over, and yet again, as much as you can bear to do it, and you will get good at it. And then, in its full scope, you'll see it. It likely won't last, this vision or this understanding, it can't last, but this is love, this is the original love or something close to it, and you'll remember it, you'll know suddenly that the grief can pass, that the rage can fade away, that you can step inside the capsule of a single moment and glimpse the calm and clarity of paradise. And when you have that, you can give it to someone else, with love; you can give it away (when people allow you to give it), yet lose nothing; you can give it over and over, give it as much as you can. When I was younger, I thought it would cost me something, I thought it would drain me, diminish me, but I was wrong. Love is infinite and divisible, and my greatest regrets are the moments I was not giving it sufficiently to you.

The editing of "Final Instructions for My Disposal"
by Vince Passaro
Edited by Jennifer Alise Drew

The following text is a composite of several drafts and sets of edits that Drew and Passaro made during their collaboration on the story. This case presents a challenge in that several different drafts that went back and forth between the author and the editor each contain different sets of edits. The files we received were labeled as pre-edit versions, that is, versions with more comments than edits, which was followed by several rounds of "edited" drafts. This is largely due to the fact that both are not only concerned with line editing but getting the best possible form for the content Passaro is working with.

As the main text, we have used an early draft where Drew is offering both comments and edits, but we have inserted some of the edits that would come up in the later drafts. Since the process involved redrafting for the sake of improving the story as such and not just smaller tweaks, it is important to showcase those changes. In the text below, you can see both the older and the revised text and some of the editor's and author's (old and new) comments. For instance, in the first sentence, Drew points out that the word "beloved" is a cliché. Subsequently, the word does not appear in any of the following drafts, and is therefore marked with strike-through. The changed text is marked in bold letters and the comments and suggested changes are put within square brackets.

Furthermore, we have used a different font and bold letters for the text that was added in one of the later drafts. For instance, when Drew objects to "a great fat-spitting fire," Passaro changes it to "send me to the fires." Some things are explained in footnotes as well. The text presented here does not, in other words, present a diachronically accurate rendition of the editing process but seeks to highlight an important range of changes to give you a sense of the attitudes of the author and the editor.

To my [beloved] [cliché] children, to beautiful[1] N__, to a few other people who shall for now remain nameless – maybe later I'll be able to name you, but currently it requires more in the way of moral resources than I have on hand.

Hear ye.

We exist physically at the molecular level; we are comprehensible as strings of protein; so, when it comes to my "remains" as they are called, for Christ's sake, just get on with it **[and burn me up in a great fat-spitting fire] [this could be better, especially given the title] send me to the fires**. I'm fifty-four now, with gray hair and gray beard, neatly trimmed for the most youthful effect a gray beard can have, and, to further express my youthful inner self-state **[what do you**

---

1   Although Drew did not object to this, the word "beautiful" was removed in the following draft, which indicates that Passaro is more attentive to, or cautious about potentially clichéd diction etc.

think about switching these hyphens? Or cutting "state"?] – a brand new baby boy; [~~I mean, he's almost three, but that's pretty new to me~~] [**also feels clichéd**]. I have also a trio of grown boys and a wonderful partner and amid this familial plenty I realize again as I have many times before that I have never written down what I want done with me, or made known my wishes regarding tubes in and hoses out, or instructed anyone where to put my meager collection of stuff, my items, the things that might be of interest or stir desire. [**I think, in keeping with a last will, you should address your boys throughout rather than at any point telling us about them – there is something that feels lacking in power in the intro here, and I think this may fix it – something to this effect:** *As I write this, I am fifty-four, with gray hair and gray beard, neatly trimmed for the most youthful effect a gray beard can have, and, to further express my youthful inner state, a baby boy – J., you have just turned three. To you and my grown boys A, B, and C, I make known my wishes regarding tubes in and hoses out, where to put my meager collection of stuff, my items . . .*]

Cash I assume there'll be none of – you know me – but I'll mention it later just in case.[2]

We exist physically at the molecular level; we are comprehensible as strings of protein; so, when it comes to my "remains" as they are called, for Christ's sake, just get on with it, send me to the fires. I'm fifty-four now, with gray hair and gray beard, neatly trimmed for the most youthful effect a gray beard can have, and, to further express my youthful inner self-state – the newest of you, a three-year-old boy who speaks of me in generally positive tones. [[He's]] [**You're?**] too young for this, [[it's meant for the rest of you]] [**This sentence throws me, partly because the "this," you're too young for this, could refer to the will, or it could refer to speaking of you in something other than positive tones? – but mostly I felt you would also be addressing this tender young lad, including him in the later "Let me tell you that I love you; and that I admire you," etc.**], really, my three grown sons and my wonderful partner. [[I realize again as I have many times before that I have never written down what I want done with me]] [**this I also want cut – too banal in an otherwise extraordinary piece**], or made known my wishes regarding tubes in and hoses out, or instructed you on how to divide my meager collection of stuff, my items, the things that might be of interest or stir desire. Cash I assume there'll be none of – you know me – but I'll mention it later just in case.[3]

Put my ashes in a silver Illy can. I prefer the espresso grind with the black stripe. You can bury it in the yard, if we ever manage to have a yard. Or, take it out to sea. I always had a distant and lazy fondness for the sea – **if you remember anything about me, you may remember that** [**Or something – to whom this is**

---

2   The following draft introduced a section break here.
3   This is an example of how Passaro rewrote the passage Drew commented on and what comments he received on the next draft.

addressed should feel consistent. It loses power when it wavers and we lose the sense of the voice speaking to these people in particular, which informs the things he says and how he confesses, shies away, circles back. You only veer away in the beginning, so it's an easy fix.] I read a lot of Conrad, not to mention Melville. Not to mention Hornblower for that matter, or Nordhoff and Hall, and all those stories of American pirates running the British blockades off the coast of New England in 1812. [I absolutely adored boats when I was young.] **[ditto here]**

But maybe you'd like to do ~~Maybe~~ something more literary. Hire some grad student to spread the ashes discreetly here and there around Flannery O'Connor's farm in Milledgeville, which is open to the public now. I am what I am, or was what I was, to the extent I ever managed to be it, because of her.

Or – here's what I'd like best, actually – take the Illy can to 1020, the **bar** at that address on Amsterdam Avenue at the corner of 110th Street, and put ~~them~~ **[it]** on the **bar** in the front corner where the painter, George the Czech, usually sits (he'll approve – if he's not in Venezuela where he spends half the year with his twenty-five-year-old mestizo girlfriend and new baby, about whom for many years his divorced wife and teenage children in New York knew not a thing). Take me there and set me up with a Jameson's straight up, a cold lager, a notebook, a Waterman, a 2B drawing pencil, a pack of Lucky Strikes, and a Leica CL. Use your iPhones to take pictures of this tableau. Send the images to all my friends. **[great]**

> *Memories of booze and expanded time and the tea-gold light through the front windows of the bars I've known on empty afternoons. No more alcohol for me you know. Oh what a story that is. Except it isn't. It's just a small unpleasant forgettable sequence, the kind that passes briefly through your mind when you're stepping over a dirty raincoat someone has abandoned on the sidewalk. Whatever the story is, you don't actually want to know it.* **[great]**

[and now we really get cooking]

The main point: once you have the ashes, whichever of you takes them from the blue-veined hands of the undertaker, do not leave them sitting around and you feeling all guilty because you haven't done something suitable with them. If you leave them sitting around then just *do* that. Move them from one closet to another every decade or so until you die. The main thing is don't feel guilty. Move on. Memory will speak what it speaks. Memory is the eternity we sometimes wish for. It has enormous vacancies in it, just like the universe – these are the collapsed black gravitational centers of longing. **[beautiful]** It's malleable, as would be any narrative taking place outside time; it, or parts of it, can happen over and over, and each time, even with different outcomes, all the contingencies remain intact – I wish I'd been able to see this earlier. Even now, I wish I could keep it in my head. Uncountable alternate universes full of the choices that, in this universe, no one made. But this is just the kind of hey-the-present-lasts-forever momentary revelation you cannot, by virtue of being human, keep in your head. Because, hello, here is life: you still have to sit on hold with the fucking insurance company. You still have to go to CVS and face Drugstore World, where language seems no longer to function as elsewhere, where no one ever understands what the fuck you're asking for. The products they sell? Never heard of them. Customers? Never heard of them. You still – in other words – have to deal with the daily matrix of enslaving bureaucracies, the enormous exhausting relentless forces that destroy meaning. All wisdom vanishes. That's the point. If you could touch the immanent God in every aspect of the universe, if you could see God and talk to God – and that is what an infinite awareness would entail – would you say hold on, I have to do my taxes? Wait, I have to deal with these fucking e-mails, let me get back to you this afternoon? Would you go to work? Would you come home? No. Wrapped in the divine, you would howl on the sidewalks naked and grab people wild-eyed, you would be picked up and taken to Bellevue, you would starve, your teeth would fall out – you would die. God is the sun, life is the glass: you're the ant. **[fantastic]**

If none of the above works for you, just spread me out around one of the elms in Riverside Park, north of 105th and south of 116th, if you can manage it, or down on the softball fields near there, by the highway and the river, where Richard Hart and Tom Adams (two sons of New Orleans) and I used to play every Thursday and Friday over the summer of 1980, after late breakfast at The Mill Luncheonette, because none of us had all that much to do – there was a paralyzing recession on, but life was cheap and I remember these as long days of freedom, in fact I remember specifically enjoying them as such, noting the freedom, tasting it as if it were a grandmother's famous sauce, as if I already knew its hours were numbered. Occasionally in those pick-up games I hit the ball off the high wall in left **[field?]**, sometimes halfway up, only twice did I see anyone hit it over, up onto the promenade – anyway, if I'm there, and you ever feel the need to come back and visit, you'll know where to go. Be done with it in any case. I won't care. By then I'll be wherever it is I'm supposed to be. If you can, pray for me. I have for you.

*   *   *

But I've gotten ahead of myself. When I'm going out – the awful part, the part with various terrifying and disgusting smells and the need for professionals just to clean up – revive me if it's worthwhile, don't if it's not. I'm sorry I can't be more specific than that but it's all I can say about it really. If you make the wrong decision, don't worry, it's not a big deal, because here's one sure fact: I'm going to die at some point, sooner rather than later by the time it comes to that stage. I'd prefer to go by reason of forces other than the *fill-out-the-forms-and-sign-here* version of bureaucratized volition. (In other words: Sign here, and we'll kill your father…. Nietzsche identified the birth of tragedy but who has remarked its death? Someone has to write the companion volume, *The De-Humanizing Impossibility of Tragedy*.) If I'm in a nice coma and don't need breathing equipment, etc., just a discreet feeding tube, then leave me there, because who knows what that's all about. I might be finding something out. You never know. Caverns of silence. Charcoal darkness. Phosphorescent fish with shallow cavities where their ancestors' eyes had been. Skip the big efforts, let me lie there, no one can bother me anymore. A quick twice-weekly chat with the nurses will do. You don't have to visit. If you're worried about the solitude, hour upon hour upon hour of it, don't. I never worry about solitude. If you're still worried, tell the nurses to use my room to sneak off and smoke cigarettes or dip snuff or drink vodka or whatever other illicit shit they might like to do, perhaps they need just a simple place to gather and complain about the others. To play rummy. To fondle **[themselves? something missing here? hard to see how you might object to this scenario though]**, or worse, their colleagues. Tell them I smile upon them. Tell them I'm happy for them. I'll enjoy the conversation. All those accents. They'll all be saying to each other *forget it* all the time. "Forget it girl, it won't never be no different," and that last will have all three of its God-given syllables . . . *Won't never be no diff-er-ahnt.* **[great]**

If you do visit – please sing. You all have such beautiful, such amazing voices.

> *The boy – fifth grade, or sixth, 12 years old, stands before the choir in the apse of the great cathedral, on which low central ground, but for the highest masses, the weekly altar is laid. He sings a Magnificat, "My soul . . . doth magnify the lord," in a voice pure and powerful. A high G of piercing beauty. He does not want to be there. His life is a series of oppressions: home, school, choir. He has perfect pitch. His talents, his skills, his various forms of brilliance daily conspire to punish him. He has a flawless calm before the crowd. He sings, perfectly, as once, much younger, eight or nine, he had played a Bach piece for violin, perfectly, at just that fine edge of perfection which can still a room. After: no elation. This is what you expect?* [Okay. Here.] [*Cut this? I can't decide.*][4]

Death, unconsciousness, stands as relief from the harrowing memories of failure, of humiliation: think of it, these things will be lifted from me, and someday too from you, as when the beautiful hostess takes your coat at a restaurant and smiles.

My funeral arrangements: now, about this, I have to say I'm feeling somewhat particular. Invite all the women. I'm serious. I want them all beckoned – some of them will come – going back to college days. Or, no: grade school. I want a large venue, many speakers; I want you strongly to encourage the comic, the inappropriate, the nakedly sentimental. Invite the hostile: *You know, I have to say, he annoyed the shit out of me.* There are some people who *really* hate me. Invite them to speak. Certain ~~very~~ successful writers of sodden forgettable sentences. Let them have at me. That'll wake people up. *What a lazy, deluded, superior, pompous fucktard. I hated the fucking guy. Glib and lazy. What did he ever do? I won the Pulitzer Prize for Christ's sake, what did he win?* I want lots of music. I want everyone to sit there and listen to all 32 minutes of "Mountain Jam," from [*Allman Brothers Live at Fillmore East*] **[okay so technically the name of the album is** *The Allman Brothers Band at*

---

4 Note: Passaro rejected this suggestion, for instance.

Fillmore East – but you can set this as referring to the show itself if you don't want to set it that way? Or we can pretend I never looked it up]. Tell people to bring drugs. Make it a party. Everyone should take some ecstasy. X. In our day it had four letters – MDCP? – something like that – **[I think what you're looking for is MDMA, unless this is meant to be a deliberate approximation?]**. Pass some joints around. Open bar in the rear two corners . . . I suppose such things cannot happen anymore. Someone, before the day is over, at least one poor schmuck whom everyone will later ridicule, should drunkenly insist on a return to freedom. Just for the hell of it.

* * *

So: I brought up the women. There are things I want you to know, but not really. I want you to glimpse the silhouette of a few things, that's all. What do any of us want to say in the end? I lived. I walked the planet. I made a few amusing remarks. I was loved.

And let it be **known**: I loved them all. Andrea (who was **known**, without irony, as Cookie), and Anna, and Ruth, and Gabrielle, and Laura, and Laureen and also a Lorene which makes no sense but she was from Dallas; Maureen Noreen Cynthia Dierdre **[Deirdre?]** Cathy Katherine Annaliese Karen Susan. Two Susan's actually. A Jenn, two n's, who knows why. I never asked. Alex, Alison, Oleh. Two Amandas and two Joannas. Two Victorias.

Tonight I'm at the counter, peeling fava beans, thinking of Debra Kelly. First love. Third grade. I was almost sick to my stomach every day. I was ill with it, literally. She ended up studying in Maine and becoming a dancer, which makes sense, one thinks of the way she stood there; her shoulders straight and her yellow hair clipped on each side and fanned across her back which curved inward toward the base of the spine, not a sway-backed curve just a subtle perfect line; and the plaid catholic school skirt centered and holding there on her hips though she was always thin, and then – but what? We were eight years old? Nine? I couldn't take my eyes away from her, except I had to or I'd start to dissolve like a lump of powdered soap under a faucet. Her skin was pale and softly defined and utterly unblemished. I decided to write a long note to Mrs. Bross, our teacher, a large woman with a stiff short hairdo the color of gold spray paint, an imposing bosom that stuck out like a shelf, and much, much perfume. Generally stern, she was most kind to me on several fraught occasions, and shocked me once with an iron hug from the desk after calling me up to the front and announcing some score I'd gotten on a standardized test. So I wrote this long note – Well, first I asked my mother what it was like, to be in love, and she started quizzing me with altogether too much amusement, so instead I wrote a long note to Mrs. Bross – asking to be transferred to the other third grade class because I just couldn't concentrate . . . This had been going on for at least four or five days. Maybe more. Maybe close to two weeks! Such a sweet slow annihilation. Oh my god, I could not believe how good this form of torment could feel. But then – wisdom – I decided to ride it out and not give Mrs. Bross that note, which would have been one of those childhood social missteps, a knife in the memory that one regrets right into the grave. I have enough of those already. But this Kelly and I were in a crowd later, in high school, or, rather, she occasionally deigned to join our crowd for a movie or a party, and talking to her remained a matter of taking my palpitating venous sense of identity into my hands and squishing it. (You can imagine the sound.) She was the only tall blonde woman I ever loved.

The next year came Maureen Pappianous. Gleaming black hair. While playing one day in the basement of her apartment building, she was burned badly by a hot water pipe breaking; she was a dark sparkling girl, shy, and kind, ever after with scarred skin over her lower neck and shoulder and arm and probably parts of her side and back and who knows where else. She was intensely beautiful, half Irish half Greek; tonight, thinking of her, it all dovetails nicely, the 10-year-old's built-in knowledge of enormous shapeless impossibility, and the later version, the midlife, hard-bordered, supremely familiar impossibility: time don't go that way brother. The sense of nostalgia and loss — all this makes a fine piece of furniture for the spirit. At such moments one knows one is alive. I sat behind her (blessed alphabet); I liked to touch her hair, ever so lightly, touching a part of her but she couldn't feel it. I did accents of the world. She and the girl beside me — whom I can't remember at all, name, face, nothing — loved this; they would request countries and I would do them. All imitations from the 4:30 movies. They could have flummoxed me so easily, what did I know of the world? They could have said Hungary or Tibet or Thailand, but of course they were no more sophisticated than I was — it was fourth grade after all — nor, it occurs to me, did they want me to fail.

Boys, see, we men, we want each other to fail, it's wired in, you fail, I succeed. But the girls don't want us to fail. This is something that men don't realize, especially after all the cruelties and rejections of adolescence: women would prefer we succeed and will help us to do so, as long as we don't catch them at it.

[Well, not all women.] **[this is absolutely necessary, but it feels expected; reword somehow, if you can think of it? I can't]**

[why in Italics? I think I liked it better in Roman, since this is your last will, and she is part of it; the Italics make it feel like a story, like one of the interludes, which it is not] *To my ex-wife I leave a list of ragged questions: Why did we do that to each other? And to our children?* ~~*What were we thinking?*~~ *Did we believe that we and they would just somehow survive all that violence? I remember only the color red. The rage and blood and your wild, murderous eyes.*

Leave your answers with my attorney. He will lock them in a file for fifty years and then they will be destroyed.

I grew up alone with [two women] **[it's far past my bedtime but am I missing something here? is this meant to address your mother or is there someone not mentioned?]**. I've watched women my whole life and I am captured by them still — I'm old, but it turns out I'm *still* not over the worst of it — the way they move, certain gestures, how they twist around to see the backs of their legs **[I see N. in this gesture, and perhaps because of what comes later**

in the hotel room, I want some moment attributed to N. here, not for her sake, though perhaps that's subconsciously so, but because she's mentioned in sentence 1 and then not again, not by name, though the section below with the bedtime ritual and the Kitchen Aid is her, and I assume the reader knows that, though perhaps not for certain]; the way they tilt their heads back slightly to put on makeup; the way they put a hand up – not all do this, but many – while they're chewing, even if they're not talking or laughing and their lips are closed. My mother (aha! you say; well, fuck you, aha yourself) sitting with her legs crossed, putting on lipstick or smoking a cigarette or sipping cold whiskey that looked brown and clear as a mountain stream – the ice made a sound like money in the glass. Her hands, small and slender and white. She smoked filterless Raleigh cigarettes and would from time to time pick a bit of tobacco from her lips or from the tip of her tongue, a gesture redolent of adulthood and sexuality. Ah, they fuck you up. It got a lot worse than that, too – I mean that kind of thing is child's play compared to what came later. There are things I haven't told you and likely won't – you would not feel enlightened by it and, really, the details don't matter: it was a complex, impacted, damaging relationship; I had a simpler but just as damaging relationship with my old man. Of course being grown up entails the long struggle to decide to try to get over it. But first we must reenact, over and over, until we know it, until we can *see* the thing: the outline of the dragon. **[all this, beautiful]**

The universe is a tongue of fire. **[ahhh -- cut this]**

He stands in the kitchen in the evening, listening to her put their boy to bed; he is rinsing a plate in soft running water and there washes over him a sense of the extraordinary privilege of the moment, her love of their child, the ease of their gracious apartment and their Kitchen Aid dishwasher which they use every day, after eating their fill, every day. Behind this thought crouches an abiding fear: that it is, all of it, undeserved, that it is unfair, that it will be taken away.

Him: that's me. But it's also not. This scene never happened. We don't have a Kitchen Aid dishwasher, that's pure fantasy; we detest the cheap dishwasher we do in fact have, which came with the place and which is growing some sort of intractable mold around the base of the inner chamber. I'm often at the sink while she is putting our boy to bed but this particular moment of fear, notwithstanding all the moments of fear one endures through the day, this one did not happen. Yet it did happen, to me, in the fact of writing it; because to write something in fictional mode that is at least minimally convincing, paradoxically requires that one experience it, whereas this is, again paradoxically, *not* required when one writes ~~write~~ convincingly in memoir: the simple announcement at the outset that *all this really happened* lifts the obligation of flawless accuracy. One must only master the voice of memory: *In the evenings I stood at the sink and listened to her put our boy to bed, she knew his books by heart, quoted them to him while she washed him and picked up his toys.* One does not *have to* experience or re-experience that moment. In that sentence, in fact, the rituals are misordered, one could not be experiencing it while writing it; but to the reader it is convincing enough, memory is enough: the past has proved itself; the present, contingent, like fiction, has not. **[great]**

Even now, at this late date, I want you to know me. This is overbearing, I realize. **[great]**

So what is at the core of life, but love? One image, for instance: a man, my age, kissing a woman in Grand Central. She was a beautiful woman. I can't get it out of my mind. **[This could almost stand alone, without the majority of the below – but see note at the end of this section.]**

So what is at the core of life, but love? An image I cannot shake**[[, of how the search never ends, of how there's never enough]]** **[What would you think about cutting this?]**: a man, my age, kissing a woman in Grand Central. ~~If these two had been married to each other, they would not have been necking at the train station~~. **[It's not that this isn't true, but it feels unnecessary, given that the whole story below makes the same point, and it also destroys the rhythm of the paragraph.]** She was a beautiful woman. I think of it now every time I'm there, in that part of the old terminal.[5]

She was waiting for him when he came off the train; she'd arrived a day or two before from Albany where she'd been staying but he couldn't get away until the Thursday; so they met that day in the famed terminal, at the last ticket booth, which is always closed – most of them are closed now – a curiously private nook of tinted marble and cast-iron window grates in a vast and definitively public space. They stood and stared, each into the other's face. Searching, searching; a look of pleasure. Eyes alight. **Sadness** *and pleasure. This thing they had, this affair of letters and chat and a few illicit phone calls, was doomed, they'd agreed it was doomed, but here they were at another moment in which* **sadness** *is built into the fervent anticipation* **[I know this means to recall the other, but I wonder if a better word might be more accurate.]**. *They kissed. He couldn't believe her mouth,* **[it felt like home]** **[ick]**. *They kissed and he was not self-conscious though he hated to see middle-aged men kissing in public, it revolted him.* ~~*They looked at each other, held each other, kissed, looked at each other again, kissed again*~~. *It had been twenty-five years since they'd met, been introduced – by whom? – and they'd spoken then only briefly,* **[[***this was in a ratty student lounge at Columbia, a room in which he could not remember ever having been unhappy. He was second year, slightly older than most, thirty, outwardly confident, accomplished; she was young, the youngest person there, a prodigy; her father was, in their circles, a famous and successful man; and so when her name was told to him early in the semester he instantly resented her as he had resented everyone privileged and everyone successful for most of the first half of his life, an enormous waste of spirit and time.***]]** **[This is lovely but all too identifying, per later note.]** *But he noticed her, he certainly did. Hers was the kind of beauty that is connected to – is inseparable from – an immutable core, a self; her face was a little crooked and animated by a light you were bathed in the minute you engaged with her or saw her smile. She was immediately striking. She had that hair. She had those* **sad** *vivid mischievous eyes. She was not that tall and neither thin nor heavy, solid, rounded, voluptuous, with sturdy limbs. They might have seen each other once or twice after that but neither remembered anything but that first meeting, brief, compelling. He felt he could remember*

---

5 Passaro followed the suggestion to make it a stand-alone passage, and here we see Drew's edit of the new version.

what she was wearing, jeans and some kind of white blouse ~~that he liked~~. She told him ~~later~~ that she'd seen him and thought, I'd like to sleep with him.

~~So there they were, in a hotel in New York, named after an exotic mammal of the Serengeti. It was expensive and thoroughly adequate. He took her first to lunch: a place they'd both known many years earlier but not together (for they had met only that one time, and not known each other after, not remained in touch through her young adulthood of fearful ambitions) and now they sat at a table of her selection; she told him later that she'd sat there by herself several times early in her career, having lunch alone, reading.~~

And then the hotel. Hours. Hours and hours. They spent much energy heaving aside the pillows, which were the size of Labradors and kept getting in the way: except then suddenly she'd grab one, with urgency and impassioned expertise, and place it beneath her in just the right way to ease some conundrum they were working through; and when this happened he thought about how accustomed she was to this. She'd told him as much. She was all about the fucking. She liked everything about it. He watched her desire, studied it; he had trouble believing in it, but there it was, undeniable. She was in an open marriage. Mainly she dated younger men: they had, she'd said archly, a certain vigor. This irritated him, of course. [In a pleasant way.] [cut?] His irritation made her glad and he knew it would make her glad so it made him glad too. ~~So~~ Later ~~here they were, fucking, and~~ he was over her and she began using her muscles to grip him — hard, really hard — and he looked at her and said I didn't know you knew how to do that and she laughed and said well I'm glad you can feel it, the 28-year-olds never seem to notice . . . He had never felt so at ease with someone new: all his life. They used condoms. Even this didn't bother him though normally it would. He couldn't come but he didn't mind because it meant they could fuck more. After every respite a new condom. It was comical, the wrappers dropped around the big bed. The vulgarity of condom wrappers on hotel floors.

[[He returned to her the next day, a little after noon, they met in the park but didn't spend much time there, walked to 33rd Street and ate a Korean lunch and then she wanted a good coffee so they found a café and she ordered cheesecake and it was excellent cheesecake even he had to admit though he'd abandoned cheesecake as a good idea many decades before. She lived far out in the upper Western corner of the nation where it rained all the time and she missed New York, where she'd grown up. It was a large issue for her; it was part of why she was there with him, these days before she returned home from her long trip East. This was New York and he was New York in every way, for her: you know you speak my mother tongue, she said to him at one point. Except it's my father tongue. Many things he said to her and wrote to her reminded her of things her father — who was not kind — would have said, did say. The man learned what these were and tried to weed them from his conversation but it was difficult, these were essential aspects of who he was and of course part of his appeal: but she didn't want to be reminded of what she was up to.]] [cut?]

[[He returned to her the next day, a little after noon, they met in the park but didn't spend much time there, walked to 33rd Street and ate a Korean lunch and then she wanted a good coffee so they found a café and she ordered cheesecake and it was excellent cheesecake even he had to admit though he'd abandoned cheesecake as a good idea many decades before. But she was in New York, she wanted cheesecake.]] [I'd still cut this.][6]

---

6 An example of a passage Passaro rewrote though Drew suggested cutting, and here we
   see she still finds it unnecessary.

She told him later – a week or two after she got home – that she had a memory, she was dropping her kids somewhere, to hip hop dance class or aikido or lacrosse; she said they parked and before anyone was out of the car in this flash moment came a sharp memory of being in bed with him and she made an involuntary sound, like ooph – but they didn't hear her. They were both boys, he wanted to say, they would never hear her in that way, but she would not believe that. A girl would have heard it instantly, would have known there was <u>something</u> **[De-emphasize? Doesn't need it.]** *in it. But not the boys. Off they went. [[She said: I drive and drive and drive. She said: This is what I do. And the laundry. There is no end to the laundry.]] [cut? Feels clichéd on second read.] She'd told him in bed on the second day that she wanted him to fuck her in the ass and he did and here, this, now, finally he was able to come, his broad peasant hand holding the headboard, slamming into her and the sounds she made – the sounds are always different when you're doing that. Of course there was lubricant on his hands so there it was, his handprint on the fabric of the headboard, which was not really a headboard but an attractive cloth-covered board attached to the wall behind the bed. Now it was like the caves in France: he had left evidence of his existence there. When she pointed it out to him he suggested he draw a deer and a figure shooting it with an arrow.*

He loved her; they loved each other; it was insane, after a couple of months of correspondence and these two days in New York, but there it was. He was ten years older than she but she was a grown woman on the cusp of middle age and neither was going to do anything foolish; yet there it was between them, a heated intimacy that was harder edged in a shared language than anything he, [with two marriages, had ever really known: they met on intellectual grounds, artistic grounds, New York grounds, moral grounds, sexual grounds; on the grounds of humor and sensibility.] [This is hard fact, too.] Later she sent him two pictures of herself as a child, small scans: she'd been one of those children who knew it all and was braving her way through, a real performer. He couldn't believe the tender beauty of her face. Her childhood, my god, it had been worse even than his own; a slaughterhouse of the spirit. Her recovery, her own marriage for its many problems and her own parenting were like the tower of glittering refuse, which, years ago, that amazing man built in Watts, a kind of imaginative miracle: People came to see it.

But of course it was all doomed; it was doomed. One day, for her, it was over.[7] ~~She fell into a depression. She couldn't talk anymore, couldn't write.~~ *Whatever this was they'd been feeling, she couldn't feel it anymore. He stopped hearing from her. He was stunned at first: no one had ever dumped him before, not unless he'd arranged it. In the first weeks he could hardly stand it: existence. It was awful.* ~~This is what grief was, he kept saying. He was supposed to feel this. Not feeling it is a mistake. He kept telling himself this. But it was awful: everything had turned noxious to him now, the light from the living room window, the window itself, the curtains, the room, the almost nauseating balmy spring air – and then sirens, far too insistent and loud for even the busiest thoroughfares of this now horrifying town. It made him sick and~~

---

7   In the new draft Passaro changed this and Drew now reacted to it, suggesting a cut: *[[But of course it was all doomed; they'd known this, said as much; it was doomed.]]* **[cut? We learn this in the first paragraph of this affair, so here it feels redundant as it only reminds me of what I knew at the outset.]**

~~then put him in pain and he felt as if every nerve ending along the surface of his skin was~~
~~mildly burning: he hurt, his whole person hurt.~~

And really it was ridiculous. He was practically an old man. Yet, for its brevity and unreality, there was something left in the wake of this intense affair that was corporal, central, undeniable – despite the pitfalls, we have to call it his heart (yes, it's a cliché, yes, his heart) – a muscle at the core of him that pushed his blood around and helped him breathe and allowed him to love and laugh and fuck and rarely, once a decade, weep – and a fresh piece of it was broken off now, **spalled,** *chipped,* ~~spalled,~~ *on the floor, lying there, and under this new light he could see not just those fragments but the poor old organ itself: it was cracked in other places and worn; and plainly its new injuries marked one more step in life, one more chunk of time, which kept moving, tumbling, rolling, skidding, toward some inevitable finish, a completion, an ending that he could not imagine, but that he knew, when it finally came, he would not fear.*

Of course, that's not me.

[This is what I do: I take other lives and for short periods weave them through my own like threads of different but complementary colors.] **[rewrite]** This is an interesting way to live; however, just as with talking with God, it keeps you from your responsibilities. **[Well this we simply don't believe, that this is not you. A few options present themselves. You could cut the whole section – it is far too long and pulls us too far outside the piece; but I know you and know you won't want to do that, and besides, you mentioned the women, and those whom you could not name at the outside of this – and without it, the piece isn't as strong, because here is the pull from the rest, here is the unknown, the pain, the stuff that necessarily drives us along but also hurts the people we're addressing the most – the impossible loves versus the possible, this only stands up as something to regret because we did not get to see it come to its own natural end, of course it wouldn't last, these things never do, but even at the ripe old age of writing last wills we still hope that it might have – so it does merit inclusion. So, you could cut the section in half, cut the unfunny part of the ending, the pain, the breakup, not necessary. I also don't like the beginning, parts of it too sentimental, the kissing, etc – and leave us the sense of the power in this relationship that you could not, did not have – very powerful, that, and the sex, great, the handprint, great, but veil it a bit more for the sake of posterity – cut Columbia, for instance. Then rewrite this last paragraph, for clearly, we know this is you.]**

There it is: don't grow old with an unblemished heart. And don't **fear** death. If you never **fear** death, you'll always be free.[8]

*   *   *

We have not yet spoken of ~~money. Or~~ the books or the cameras or the lenses or the nice art supplies and Watermen pens or the four and a half feet of old journals. Just

---

8   New version where only repetitions of "fear" are highlighted.

decide among yourselves. Anything someone wants he should have. If more than one want it, add it to a pile to be considered later; trade and barter one thing against another. Divide among you equally my reputation, such as it is, and use it as sunscreen. The language, the images, the rights, the proper disposition: projecting my consciousness forward, I can see that it will be remarkable to me and others how little interest my work will have for me when I'm dying. I shall assign a literary executor: **fear** not. To this person please deliver the journals: and don't think about them anymore. If something of them gets published, don't worry about it. After two weeks it's forgotten and really, even from the first, no one gives a shit. Secrets are a dream.

[John] **[disguise?]**: you'll remember how two or three years ago we discussed counterpoint, which you were studying formally and which I was attempting to employ, in a class, as an aesthetic model in terms of which one could understand certain conflicting literary texts. And you said: do you write like that? And I said no, I have trouble enough writing straight realistic narrative, I go completely off the rails if I try anything too unusual, and you said, isn't it painful to you that you can't do the kind of work you think so highly of? And I was startled by the question (I didn't say but ought to have said what I first thought, which was, at your age, oh yes, every great sentence I saw that I had not written pierced me in that way) but I thought about it for a second and said, no, oddly enough. The only painful thing is failing to do the work I know I *can* do. I'm very thankful when I *do* manage to do it.

It's like that: I'm glad whatever's done at the end is done – let it go; it's a plastic bag in the wind over the West Side Highway. It will land somewhere. (Probably on a window ledge at the New York Psychiatric Center at 168th Street. [Don't go fetch it. These are not the window ledges for you.] **[Cut these last 2 lines?]**)[9]

There is no money, that's the upshot. You certainly won't be surprised. I have a nice insurance policy at work, a hefty sum if there were only one of you, but divided four ways it is more like part of a down payment on a house. Maybe. Anyway there's that. Try to be happy.

*(If you're interested in money, each of you is quite sufficiently smart to make plenty of it. Only self-consciousness and various moral considerations and perhaps aesthetic and cultural distaste stand in the way of amassing large sums of money. [And] **[But?]** if money is what you want, all these impediments, moral, aesthetic, blah blah, can be jettisoned.* ~~*Watch the others. Do what they do.*~~ *I don't ever remember meeting someone who was very rich and also imaginative. Just imitate.)* **[I wonder, since this is not in the same vein as the other italicized portions, if this ought to be put in Roman and not offset. What do you think? The parentheses are strong enough without the rest, I think.] [Passaro's answer: I want to keep the parens. I've pulled out the space breaks which should be reserved – or I've tried to reserve them – for the spots that also merit the little do-dads.]**

---

9   These two paragraphs were cut in the following draft.

In the end, if only each of us was able to enjoy his own existence, as those who've loved us enjoyed us. Let me try to give you that, since as of now, it's clear, I have little else to give you. Let me tell you that I love you; and that I admire you. That you have **sharp** minds, sharp tongues, and, best of all, sharp **[these sharps are great; change the below]** consciences. You love the woods. You can make music. You understand complex numbers and simple machines. You are kind to children. You believe there is beauty in the world, and you pursue it and share it.

[Drew: space break here? or no?] [Passaro: yes.]

Well boys let me disclose the gifts reserved for age. Self-forgiveness comes on slowly but **sharply**, like a recurring memory of incomprehensible joy. The treasures of solitude are best enjoyed in youth; I have come to recognize that my drive for solitude, in middle life and beyond, is a poisonous addiction. To seek others and then to push them away is, first of all, mean and unfair; but for you, if you're the one doing it, it's like rowing one way with the left arm, the other way with the right. Having gotten nowhere and gained nothing, you're still exhausted.

I **realized** something last year when I was going to be best man at the wedding of my friend [Josh and his bride, Elizabeth] **[disguise? T.]** came, as did I, from an unstable and ultimately shattered set of circumstances. Nevertheless he has made himself into a funny, generous, kind, and only mildly neurotic adult. His wedding took place downtown not far from the site of the World Trade Center. And over the days before the wedding, as I compressed various thoughts, a process that would lead me to be able to make a toast, I **realized** that in recent years I've come to know some young people, decent, smart, talented, likeable, from very stable and prosperous homes, and in knowing them I became aware of the basic position of security upon which they stood to face the world: you guys mostly don't have it, **[It strikes me now that this wouldn't be true of Jonah, and it may strike the reader as an oversight, since the 3-year-old you mention would not still be in the same circumstance of upbringing as those from the ex-wife you mention so memorably; do you think it merits clarification?][10]** I never had it, and **T.** if possible had it even less; and I **realized** at some point near the wedding that people such as **T.** and I came into our adulthoods and faced the dilemma of building strong and secure identities – in relation to the world around us, its indifference, our desires – with nothing at all supporting us; whereas some other people have very solid ground beneath them. And the image I thought of was that of Philippe Petit, who crossed between the World Trade Towers **[twin towers? Since WTC is already mentioned.]** on a high wire the year I came to New York (I was 18, recently orphaned, completely set loose in the world). The images of Petit on the wire remained vivid for me all these years, and suddenly I understood, at least in part, why: this was us, I told **T.** in the toast: hanging between those absurd and beautiful towers; Petit represented people like us, achieving our existence, our

---

10 This note was for instance made in the third draft which is when the editing itself has started and few comments were made.

sense of who we were, out there in gray light with nothing but a hundred stories of air beneath us and facing a 40-mile-an-hour wind.

Flannery O'Connor several times in her letters quoted the French (very Catholic) writer François Mauriac's advice for the artist: "Purify the source." That's a lifetime's project. The first requirement is surviving your high-wire walk to selfhood. And then, one approach might be (I certainly haven't gotten there and can't say for sure) to look toward what you want. Move toward what you want. But while you're doing that, work on wanting the right things. Never relent. After you give up, go back. Give up again, go back again. I am often slowed to a crawl by a sense that what I want to do is too hard; I'm too soft; it's not worth it; it's all futile. Then I go back.

Once we're old we can [see so clearly the dilemmas of the young] **[feels somewhat trite]**, but the advice we have to offer is rarely of any use at all. It's not even audible; it's barely coherent. [It's a cry to the drowning man, "Don't be afraid − all you need to do is swim!" This kind of advice is always true and it always misses the point − it's not even in the same hemisphere as the point.] **[Rework this and the end is brilliant -- the next long paragraph says it all, so here maybe just a bit of humor to lead us into it unawares.]**

Once we're older − very few people from middle age onward won't claim this − youth and its problems seem to scream out for our advice. It all looks so clear, so manageable to us. But the advice we have to offer is almost entirely ridiculous. Think of **[?]** *The Graduate.* A guy like Benjamin, in 1968, shit, "plastics" was unbelievably great advice. This was before the grocery bags, before the garbage bags, these were the days of Bakelite and ceramics, brass-bodied cameras and steel-bodied cars. Fucking Benjamin could have retired at fifty and traveled the world with a well-preserved Katherine Ross.[11] Advising the young is like telling a drowning man all he needs to do is swim.

Once we're older − very few people from middle age onward won't claim this − youth and its problems seem to scream out for our advice. It all looks so clear to us now, so much more manageable than it is when you're in it. ~~, so manageable to us~~. But the advice we have to offer is almost entirely ridiculous. ~~Think of [?] The Graduate. A guy like Benjamin, in 1968, shit, "plastics" was unbelievably great advice. This was before the grocery bags, before the garbage bags, these were the days of Bakelite and ceramics, brass-bodied cameras and steel-bodied cars. Fucking Benjamin could have retired at fifty~~50 ~~and traveled the world with a well-preserved Katherine Ross.~~ **[I enjoy this Graduate bit but it's exactly the wrong example: plastics was terrible advice and Benjamin attacking the church and pulling her out and grabbing a bus: that was correct. Sooo—]** It's ~~Advising the young is~~ like telling a drowning man all he needs to do is swim.[12]

Nevertheless here I go.

When people tell you they love you: listen to them.

---

11 This was the new draft of the section, rewritten after Drew made her comment.

12 In the fourth draft Passaro was still working with this passage and here we see his own rewrites, cuts, and comments.

Don't dismiss it, or think them foolish. Try to see yourself as they see you. Just for a moment. Realize the dignity you have, struggling in the world, most days with some tangible grace. Realize your courage. See the beauty, your own beauty. Do this just for a moment – you only need a moment. But do it over and over, and over and over, and yet again, as much as you can **remember** and bear to do it, and you will get good at it. And then, in its full scope, you'll see it. It won't last, this vision or this understanding, it can't last and I know it won't last, but this is love, this is the original love or something close to it, and you'll **remember** it, you'll know how the grief can pass, and the rage can fade away, and that you can step inside the capsule of a single moment and know the clarity of paradise. And when you have that, you can give it to someone else, with love; you can give it away (when people allow you to give it), yet lose nothing; you can give it over and over, give it as much as you can. When I was younger, I thought it would cost me something, it would drain me, but I was wrong. It is infinite and divisible and my greatest regrets are the moments I was not giving it sufficiently to you.

"Final Instructions for my Disposal"
Conversation with Vince Passaro and Jennifer Alise Drew

The editors

In the editing process with Vince Passaro, on his short story "Final Instructions for My Disposal," we find several different issues we would like to discuss: knowing the author, the question of address (in relation to the content), fiction v. nonfiction, clichés, sentimental prose, trite prose, cutting.

Let us begin with the working relationship. We find that your correspondence with Passaro is essential in that it conveys a certain intimacy that the editing process seems to call for, and we appreciate you sharing it with us. Can you say a few words about the way this affects the process? Would you say that this fact makes you harsher and more blunt in your commentary because you know that the author is able to take your advice on board?

Drew

When I met Vince, I was working in New York for a now-defunct magazine called *Madison*, what we aspirationally liked to call a hybrid of *Vanity Fair* and *The New Yorker*, with thicker, glossier pages and a far smaller staff. This was in 1999–2000, when paper magazines were still viable. The first time I talked to Vince I was fact-checking one of his essays or criticisms – maybe his review of *A Heartbreaking Work of Staggering Genius*, which had just come out, or the piece on Mary McCarthy that began a whole new literary awakening for me – and that conversation began our friendship. In the spring of 2002, I left the city to work with Hunter S. Thompson in Colorado: a job Vince unintentionally helped me get by putting me in touch with David Rosenthal, then publisher of Simon & Schuster, who was also Hunter's longtime editor. (Simon & Schuster published Vince's first novel, *Violence, Nudity, Adult Content*, in 2002.) The early 2000s were rather large years for both of us, and our relationship became the kind you can really only have through letters (or in our case, email) – on a different plane from those relationships you have with people you see every day. There is history there, and trust, and private knowledge, as well as much of my learning as a writer and editor. I am definitely less professional, I suppose the word might be, in how I approach the editing process with Vince; at least, I don't feel I need to be as careful with my explanations, or couch my critical comments as much. I know he can take it, would see through any attempts at veiling anyway, and will argue with me without reservation, this last of which is crucial: editing has to be a collaboration.

I would say that intimacy is part of the enterprise in general: there is some trust required on the part of the author to submit the work, and on the part of the editor to take it on: it becomes a temporary shared project, and the real work that happens, happens on a level above grammar or punctuation, or even plot and story. It's not possible to have this kind of collaboration with every writer, of course, because some writers are not open to it. And in order to get there, you can't only be critical. There is an element of necessary praise. I learned this working with Hunter: you can accomplish very little if the writer believes you aren't on his side, aren't on board with what he is trying to do.

Vince was working on that first novel when we met, and while the manuscript was with his editor at Simon & Schuster, he asked me to read it. I can still recall sitting with the pages in the tiny room I was renting at the time, from a retired ballet dancer on Manhattan's Upper West Side. I had put all my stuff in storage, and sat on my bed to work, and smoked cigarettes out a tiny window that I then had to leave open, so the bamboo blinds, too big for the window, slapped the walls with the wind (it was winter). It was not a particularly good time in my life, and reading Vince's book was a pleasure. I took notes on the brown paper bag the manuscript came in, and referred to them when I talked to Vince on the phone about one scene in the book, about eight pages, that takes place in the stall of the men's bathroom: a masturbation scene, a rather lengthy one, and while it's going on the narrator's mind wanders across a murder that occurred in his family. My first instinct was to question the scene's merit and inclusion, consider excising it – which, Vince told me later, his editor felt he should do – but I realized that it was, in a way, the soul of the project: that what may seem to be tangential and perhaps somewhat shocking is in fact what sets one writer apart from another, what distinguishes a person and his/her work from the rest. There was a kernel, or perhaps more than a kernel, of biographical truth to the story of the murder, and that taught me another lesson about the permeability, the thin skin dividing fiction and non-fiction. I've just reread that scene after fifteen, sixteen years, and am floored by it: whole worlds go by in just a few pages, all these remembered women, one in particular, the tribute to the uncle, the humor: it goes so many places and that in itself, the realism and the build, its rhythm and language, not just the sex act of course but the way it shows how we think in moments of solitude, and the description of the murder scene: really extraordinary.

Passaro

My own memory is that back at the beginning, you didn't know how authorized (funny word) you were so we'd be editing on the phone and I'd hear some doubt on your end, a pause, a roadbump of stillness, and I'd say, what is it, what's wrong, and being avid, you'd then tell me without hesitation. Eventually I had to ask less and less, but still had to sometimes, because you sensed where I might be resistant, as opposed to seeing instantly the wisdom of your ways. Fiction's also a little different from nonfiction. Fiction can make its own rules. But at this point yes, I would bet: the relationship is essential to the editing process because it is the foundation on which trust rests. What every writer fears is that the editor doesn't actually like the work, doesn't appreciate it, doesn't think particularly well of the author – or that the editor is a linguistic oaf. What every editor fears is that the writer is going to be an unreasonable nutjob who goes off at every correction and who doesn't understand basic grammar and conventions of usage. So we know each other now and yes, you can say "trite" or "cliché" (or the coup de grâce, "ick") to me, and know you can, and I'll stagger a little then staunch the wound with my handy "writer repair" kit and carry on.

The editors

What were the key areas of editorial focus for you at the point of submission?

Drew

It's inevitable, given the above, that I read Vince's work having far more knowledge of the author than will the reader, so my initial thoughts focused on modulating what I knew to be true in the story, and therefore perhaps muddied it unnecessarily; I felt protective of some of the details Vince had revealed, and wanted to stuff them back into the fictional framework of the piece. These concerns came up especially in the passage halfway through the piece, the interlude in italics that we discussed at length in revisions, which begins, "She was waiting for him when he came off the train" – this passage reminded me of the masturbation scene in his novel and I felt it functioned in a similar way. It wasn't yet where it needed to be, as the center of things, was too long and too personally revealing. But more on that below.

There was also the matter of the beginning, which seemed slow to me, slowed down by a few clichés or toss-away phrases that felt like placeholders for a later draft. Vince has said that beginnings are the most difficult, having "qualities of the overture," and this is true; I also felt there was an incompatibility between the form of address – the piece opens by addressing those for whom it's intended: "To my children, to N, to a few other people who shall for now remain nameless – maybe later I'll be able to name you, but currently it requires more in the way of moral resources than I have on hand" – and the telling that happens about the narrator's family: "I have also a trio of grown boys . . ." I wanted to let the reader work out the family details through what's said, and left, to these boys. The telling extends to some of the statements the narrator makes – "I always had a distant and lazy fondness for the sea" – a wonderful line, and the kind of thing I suppose some people never know about their parents and lovers. But that didn't feel right for this narrator; that isn't the kind of relationship he has, or wants to have, with his children, so we don't quite believe it.

But this is a tricky thing, as the reader needs to know things the intended recipients of the testament would already know. There is a very delicate balance between the two. A few lines into the story, we read:

> I'm fifty-four now, with gray hair and gray beard, neatly trimmed for the most youthful effect a gray beard can have, and, to further express my youthful self-state – every middle-aged man's accessory if he can't afford a European sports car – a young child, the newest of you, a highly enjoyable three-year-old boy who still speaks of me in generally positive terms.

This dance goes on throughout: between the narrator's writing to the people he loves, the things they do not and perhaps, he says, should not know, and his writing to himself and the rest of us, all of that which he isn't quite prepared to leave behind.

For me, on that first read-through, the piece really got going with this paragraph, a good example of the intelligence and wit and narrative grace that, along with his ear for rhythm, combine to make Vince's voice the singular thing that it is:

> The main point: once you have the ashes, whichever of you takes them from the dyshidrotic hands of the funeral director, probably not old, probably surprisingly young, the business has to have some young people in it after all, do not leave them sitting around and you feeling all guilty because you haven't done something suitable with them. If you leave them sitting around then just *do* that. Move them from one closet to another every decade or so until you die. The main thing is, don't feel guilty. Move on. Memory will speak what it speaks. Memory is the eternity we sometimes wish for. . . . Memory is malleable, as would be any narrative taking place outside time; it, or parts of it, can happen over and over, and, even with different outcomes, all the contingencies will remain intact – I wish I'd been able to see this earlier. Even now, I wish I could keep it in my head.

In the first draft, this read "the blue-veined hands of the undertaker," one of those clichés I instinctively hate, because we gloss right over descriptors like "blue-veined," being overused for hands and other parts of the body: it doesn't tell us much of interest. Vince eventually changed this to "dyshidrotic hands," which I had to look up, to verify the spelling and because I'd never seen the word. It became another phrase that occasionally runs through my mind: *dyshidrotic hands of the undertaker.* I've never forgotten it, in part because I realized that little word described the mysterious problem I was having with my own hands. Along with dyshidrotic hands and a distant and lazy fondness for the sea, I've recently discovered that Vince and I also share an olfactory phantosmia: we smell cigarette smoke where there is none (which at least in my case is pure longing for something I had to give up).

The editors

The issue of address. In your initial comments to the opening of the original draft, you write: "I think, in keeping with a last will, you should address your boys throughout rather than at any point telling us about them – there is something that feels lacking in power in the intro here." Then you go on to rewrite a segment to show what you mean. This is an excellent suggestion, which requires the editor to work with the potential of the narrative, and to trust the author to perform. Would you have accepted a "No" for an answer? As editors, we feel that some things are up for discussion, but some are requirements. Of course, until one has tried, there is no knowing how effective the suggestion may be.

Drew

I'm not sure I ever have hard requirements. Writers often say no, and sometimes I think this is a mistake, but more often these push-pull conversations are exactly what editing is about: getting a story closer to what it is meant to be. In the best case, these "no's" tell me I'm pushing in a direction that is contrary to the story: that I'm perhaps trying to make it into something I would have written or wanted to read instead of what it actually is. Of course, some writers just aren't open to changes, or to editing in general, and that's a whole different affair. In Vince's case, I think – mostly because he agreed with me – that this suggestion was the right one: again there's the compatibility and trust that allows us to work well together, but it's also emblematic of how sensitive an editor has to be in order to be any good: we have to be able to slip into the voice of the writer and think like the writer and less like a person critiquing the work.

The editors

Passaro writes to you, "Fiction must be – is required to be, if it is to work and if it is to matter – truer than nonfiction." Indeed, his story contains elements of creative nonfiction/memoir. A significant issue in the early edits concerns those lines between fact and fiction and what perhaps ought or ought not to be made public. This is partly related to you knowing the author. You write:

> Well this we simply don't believe, that this is not you. A few options present
> themselves. You could cut the whole section – it is far too long and pulls us
> too far outside the piece; but I know you and know you won't want to do that,
> and besides, you mentioned the women, and those whom you could not name

at the outset of this – and without it, the piece isn't as strong, because here is the pull from the rest, here is the unknown, the pain, the stuff that necessarily drives us along but also hurts the people we're addressing the most – the impossible loves versus the possible, this only stands up as something to regret because we did not get to see it come to its own natural end, of course it wouldn't last, these things never do, but even at the ripe old age of writing last wills we still hope that it might have – so it does merit inclusion. So, you could cut the section in half, cut the unfunny part of the ending, the pain, the breakup, not necessary … and leave us the sense of the power in this relationship that you could not, did not have – very powerful, that, and the sex, great, the handprint, great, but veil it a bit more for the sake of posterity – cut Columbia, for instance. Then rewrite this last paragraph, for clearly, we know this is you.

When you use "we" here, what do you mean? Is it mainly your knowledge of the author that makes you react to certain details, or do you feel that general audiences would have a similar reaction and feel this hits too close to the target?

In what sense is the relationship between editor and writer a "protective" one? Passaro talks of "intend[ing] to remind the reader faintly somehow that it's more me in the writing of it than in the living of it." Could you talk about particular changes that were required to achieve this, to blur those boundaries, and the impact these have on the story as a whole?

Furthermore, you are both specific about the details that you want cut and also suggest that a major cut be made by the author. You think the story would be just fine without this entire section, but sense that it has great value to the author so you do not push for its removal. We feel that your work here goes deeper than the question of what makes the story better, and this is indeed very important, but not something every editor can do with any story. This highlights how individualized our work with each piece may be and what all the different levels of engagement may be. Can you comment on all this?

Drew

I suppose I'm using "we" in two senses: "we" the reader, as in the first and last claims – *well this we simply don't believe / we know this is you* – and "we" as you and me, people driven by the same things that drive the narrator – *here is the pull from the rest, here is the unknown, the pain, the stuff that necessarily drives us along.*

As I said earlier, I felt protective of some of the personal details Vince revealed because, aside from making it easier on his people to read the thing (which is not my business, I realize, but hey, we're friends too), I didn't want these details to get in the way of where the story was going, and it felt to me a few of them were doing that: were standing in the way of the through line, or just the rhythm of the unfolding. There is, in any kind of writing, the right balance of detail to serve the story, regardless of whether you're describing a fictional or real character, and I felt, in that long, italicized section about the woman from the train, that the description of their history together was too tangential, inessential, never mind that I recognized some of Vince's own life in it. I did not, however, feel the piece would be fine without the entire section: as I wrote in that first read-through, "without it, the piece isn't as strong" – I knew when I saw it that it was one of those passages that wasn't yet where it needed to be, the locus, and we needed to whittle it down and find its core. After all, when you're writing a last will and testament (or, as in the earlier example, doing certain things in a bathroom stall), these are the things one thinks of, unbidden or otherwise: without these remembered moments, without these italic interludes, the story would be a paler version of life, of truth: it would be less believable, and certainly less strong. Or, as Vince has it, "this section had to work enough like the others for the story to maintain its tightrope walk over the maelstrom where what is written and what is true meet and collide."

This long passage is an example of how we worked. It changed quite a lot in the process, and is in fact one of the few sections that kept changing. The first version is the following:

So what is at the core of life, but love? One image, for instance: a man, my age, kissing a woman in Grand Central. She was a beautiful woman. I can't get it out of my mind. **[This could almost stand alone, without the majority of the below – but see note at the end of this section.]**
She was waiting for him when he came off the train; she'd arrived a day or two before from Albany where she'd been staying but he couldn't get away until the Thursday; so they met that day in the famed terminal, at the last ticket booth, which is always closed – most of them are closed now – a curiously private nook of tinted marble and cast-iron window grates in a vast and definitively public space. They stood and stared, each into the other's face. Searching, searching; a look of pleasure. Eyes alight. Sadness and pleasure. This thing they had, this affair of letters and chat and a few illicit phone calls, was doomed, they'd agreed it was doomed, but here they were at another moment in which sadness is built into the fervent anticipation. They kissed. He couldn't believe her mouth, [it felt like home] [ick].*They kissed and he was not self-conscious though he hated to see middle-aged men kissing in public, it revolted him. It had been twenty-five years since they'd met, been introduced – by whom? – and they'd spoken then only briefly.* [[this was in a ratty student lounge at Columbia, a room in which he could not remember ever having been unhappy. He was second year, slightly older than most, thirty, outwardly confident, accomplished; she was young, the youngest person there, a prodigy; her father was, in their circles, a famous and successful man; and so when her name was told to him early in the semester he instantly resented her as he had resented everyone privileged and everyone successful for most of the first half of his life, an enormous waste of spirit and time.]] **[This is lovely but all too identifying, per later note.]** *But he noticed her, he certainly did. Hers was the kind of beauty that is connected to – is inseparable from – an immutable core, a self; her face was a little crooked and animated by a light you were bathed in the minute you engaged with her or saw her smile. She was immediately striking. She had*

that hair. She had those sad vivid mischievous eyes. She was not that tall and neither thin nor heavy, solid, rounded, voluptuous, with sturdy limbs. They might have seen each other once or twice after that but neither remembered anything but that first meeting, brief, compelling. He felt he could remember what she was wearing, jeans and some kind of white blouse that he liked. She told him later that she'd seen him and thought, I'd like to sleep with him.

In this second version, Vince separated the sections and made some bigger changes:

So what is at the core of life, but love? An image I cannot shake, of how the search never ends, of how there's never enough: a man, my age, kissing a woman in Grand Central. ~~If these two had been married to each other, they would not have been necking at the train station.~~ *[It's not that this isn't true, but it feels unnecessary, given that the whole story below makes the same point, and it also destroys the rhythm of the paragraph.]* She was a beautiful woman. I think of it now every time I'm there, in that part of the old terminal.

She was waiting for him when he came off the train; she'd arrived a day or two before from upstate where she'd been staying but he couldn't get away until the Thursday; so they met that day in the famed terminal, at the last ticket booth, which is always closed – most of them are closed now – a curiously private nook of tinted marble and cast-iron window grates in a vast and definitively public space. They stood and stared, each into the other's face. Searching, searching; a look of pleasure. Eyes alight. Sadness and pleasure. This thing they had, this affair of letters and chat and a few illicit phone calls, was doomed, they'd agreed it was doomed, but here they were at another moment in which sadness is built into the fervent anticipation. They kissed. He couldn't believe her mouth. They kissed and he was not self-conscious, though he hated to see middle-aged men kissing in public, it revolted him. It had been twenty-five years since they'd met, been introduced – by whom? – and they'd spoken then only briefly, graduate students at the university, standing in the ratty coffee lounge, a room in which he could not remember ever having been unhappy. He was second year, slightly older than most, twenty-nine, outwardly confident, accomplished; she was young, the youngest person there, a prodigy; her father was, in their circles, a famous and successful man; and so when her name was told to him early in the semester he noticed her, he certainly did. Hers was the kind of beauty that is connected to – is inseparable from – an immutable core, a self; her face was a little crooked and animated by a light you were bathed in the minute you engaged with her or saw her smile. She was immediately striking. She had that hair. She had those sad vivid mischievous eyes. She was not that tall and neither thin nor heavy, solid, rounded, voluptuous, with sturdy limbs. They might have seen each other once or twice after that but neither remembered anything but that first meeting, brief, compelling. He felt he could remember what she was wearing, jeans and some kind of white blouse ~~that he liked~~. She told him ~~later~~ that she'd seen him and thought, I'd like to sleep with him.

In this third installment, the passage is still in progress:

> So what is at the core of life, but love? An image I cannot shake**[[, of how the search never ends, of how there's never enough]]** *[What would you think about cutting this?]*: a man, my age, kissing a woman in Grand Central. She was a beautiful woman. I think of it now every time I'm there, in that part of the station.
>
> *She was waiting for him when he came off the train; she'd arrived a day or two before from upstate, where she'd been staying, but he couldn't get away until the Thursday; so they met that day in the famed terminal, at the last ticket booth, which is always closed — most of them are closed now — a curiously private nook of tinted marble and cast-iron window grates in a vast and definitively public space. They stood and stared, searching; a look of pleasure. Eyes alight.* **Sadness** *and pleasure. This thing they had, this affair of letters* **[?]** *and a few illicit phone calls, was doomed, they'd agreed it was doomed, but here they were at another moment in which* **sadness [I know this means to recall the other, but I wonder if a better word might be more accurate.]** *is built into the fervent anticipation. They kissed. He couldn't believe her mouth. It had been twenty-five years since they'd met, been introduced — by whom? — and they'd spoken then only briefly, graduate students at the university, standing in the ratty coffee lounge, a room in which he could not remember ever having been unhappy. He was second-year, slightly older than most, twenty-nine, outwardly confident, accomplished; she was young, the youngest person there, a prodigy. Hers was the kind of beauty that is connected to — is inseparable from — an immutable core, a self; her face was a little crooked and animated by a light you were bathed in the minute you engaged with her or saw her smile. She was immediately striking. She had that hair. She had those* **sad** *vivid mischievous eyes. She was not that tall and neither thin nor heavy, solid, rounded, voluptuous, with sturdy limbs. They might have seen each other once or twice again but neither remembered anything except that first meeting, brief, compelling. She told him that she'd seen him and thought, I'd like to sleep with him.*

In the final version, it reads:

> So, what is at the core of life but love? An image I cannot shake: a man, my age, kissing a woman in Grand Central. She was a beautiful woman. I think of it now every time I'm there, in that part of the station.
>
> *She was waiting for him when he came off the train; she'd arrived a day or two before from upstate, where she'd been staying, but he couldn't get away until the Thursday; so they met that day in the famed terminal, at the last ticket booth, which is always closed — most of them are closed now — a curiously private nook of tinted marble and cast-iron window grates in a vast and definitively public space. They stood and stared, searching; a look of pleasure. Eyes alight. Sadness and pleasure. This thing they had, this affair of letters and a few illicit phone calls, was doomed, they'd agreed it was doomed, but here they were at another moment in which loss is built into the fervent*

anticipation. They kissed. He couldn't believe her mouth. It had been twenty-five years since they'd met, been introduced – by whom? – and they'd spoken then only briefly, graduate students at the university, standing in the ratty coffee lounge, a room in which he could not remember ever having been unhappy. He was second-year, slightly older than most, twenty-nine, outwardly confident, accomplished; she was young, the youngest person there, a prodigy. Hers was the kind of beauty that is connected to – is inseparable from – an immutable core, a self; her face was a little crooked and animated by a light you were bathed in the minute you engaged with her or saw her smile. She was immediately striking. She had that hair. She had those sad vivid mischievous eyes. She was not that tall and neither thin nor heavy; she was solid, rounded, sturdy, voluptuous. She was not one whose fire needed to be lit; it was burning already. They might have seen each other once or twice again after that, but neither remembered anything except the first meeting, brief, compelling. She told him that she'd seen him and thought, I'd like to sleep with him.

The editors

Within the editing process there is a lengthy debate over what appear to be fairly small, sentence-level issues – the text is closely dissected to examine rhythms and weightings (and in some great detail, even the presence of certain commas) – and more than this, something that perhaps can't be easily quantified: the (emotive) impact of syntactical changes on semantic meaning. For example, the final lines of Passaro's story are these: "When I was younger, I thought it would cost me something, I thought it would drain me, diminish me, but I was wrong. Love is infinite and divisible, and my greatest regrets are the moments I was not giving it sufficiently to you."

Passaro: "Last line of the piece should be revised to read: 'Love is infinite and divisible, and my greatest regrets TK TK the moments I was not giving it sufficiently to you.' [sic] Here I need some advice. I don't like 'are the moments' because it's weak and inaccurate: the regrets are not the moments. So 'my greatest regrets arise from the moments?' abide in the moments? reside in the moments?"

Drew: "Love is infinite and divisible, and my greatest regrets are the moments I wasn't giving it sufficiently to you – is it too pedestrian to suggest Love is infinite and divisible, and my greatest regret is not giving it sufficiently to you? The moments add something, after the rest of that paragraph and its emphasis on moments, but maybe there again you don't need the moments after all? Though I also hate to lose regrets plural, if that is how one thinks of it. My greatest regrets are not giving it sufficiently?"

Passaro: "Actually how about this – just occurred to me: 'Love is infinite and divisible, and what I regret most are the moments I was not giving it sufficiently to you.' ?

No. '. . . and my greatest regrets come from the moments I was not giving it sufficiently to you.' either that or 'arise from the moments.'

What do you think, between those two?"

Could you talk to us about why these details were so important to get right? How did the changes affect the tone of the story, particularly given that these are the lines with which the reader departs the narrative?

Drew

Syntax has everything to do with meaning: some of my greatest regrets as both a writer and editor are about the smallest things, having chosen to go with one word over another: there is an acre of difference between "I" and "our," or between "our" and "your," for example, and what one chooses hangs over the rest. This might be a good example of where editing can go south; while it may be true that regrets are not moments, while it may be more accurate to say "what I regret are the moments," that revision falls flat on the page, and these statements aren't so far from each other as they sound. What Vince ended up with was very nearly the same thing with which he began – in the very first draft he sent me, the last line read:

> It is infinite and divisible and my greatest regrets are the moments I was not giving it sufficiently to you.

The final copy reads:

> Love is infinite and divisible, and my greatest regrets are the moments I was not giving it sufficiently to you.

As I said before, Vince is good at endings. He had to go through a few iterations, perhaps, in order to confirm the truth of the thing. But you can see where the comma and the clear antecedent make the difference.

The editors

Your sensitivity to clichés, sentimentality, and triteness is great. In one place you attack one of the clichés in the later drafts, but otherwise you go straight at it from the first sets of comments. Some instances:

1. To my **[beloved]** [*cliché*] children,
2. a brand-new baby boy **[I mean, he's almost three, but that's pretty new to me.]** [*also feels clichéd*],
3. Once we're old we can **[see so clearly the dilemmas of the young]** [*feels somewhat trite*],
4. You write: "I also don't like the beginning, parts of it too sentimental, the kissing",
5. The universe is a tongue of fire. [*ahhh – cut this*]

Can you say a few words about these issues?

Drew

I owe some of this sensitivity to Leslie Epstein, former director of Boston University's graduate creative writing program; he still held that position when I was there.

Leslie has a hatred of overwriting, in particular: echoes; using more than one simile or metaphor on a page; and clichés. I agree with him about the echoes and the clichés. He felt strongly enough, and probably wearied of saying it for thirty-plus years, that he handed out a "tip sheet" of rules to all his students (and may still). This line has stuck with me: "while not doing too much violence to your natural style, try to use as few adjectives and especially adverbs as possible." Those "while not" and "try to" are generous allowances for certain dead and accomplished writers, but generally, I've found his advice to be sound. (Leslie, by the way, is reputed to have broken many a writer; I happen to be grateful to him for breaking me of my bad habits, sentimentality in particular. But then I suppose, on the heels of Hunter Thompson, Leslie didn't scare me as much as maybe he should. I'll leave in that "broken/breaking" echo just for him.) But really, the most important part of Leslie's advice, the part that still plays through my mind, is about "not doing too much violence to your natural style," or really any at all: that is the key, of course – the world only needs one Raymond Carver.

The truth is, there's no good reason to have three "likes" in a paragraph just as there's no good reason to submit to ordinary, inexact phrases, especially those that have been used so much they no longer hold much meaning – and about that "tongue of fire," I suppose there's the other bit of advice about not using pound words when shilling words will do, or removing the flashy bits to say something more grounded. John McPhee wrote an essay in *The New Yorker* a few years ago ("Draft No. 4") in which, among other things, he advocates for using the dictionary in revisions – to sit there with our drafts until we find what stands behind those placeholder words, what we are trying to say that is different from what has been said before. He writes,

> You draw a box not only around any word that does not seem quite right but also around words that fulfill their assignment but seem to present an opportunity. While the word inside the box may be perfectly O.K., there is likely to be an even better word for this situation, a word right smack on the button, and why don't you try to find such a word? . . . If there's a box around "sensitive," because it seems pretentious in the context, try "susceptible." Why "susceptible"? Because you looked up "sensitive" in the dictionary and it said "highly susceptible." With dictionaries, I spend a great deal more time looking up words I know than words I have never heard of – at least ninety-nine to one. The dictionary definitions of words you are trying to replace are far more likely to help you out than a scattershot word from a thesaurus. . . . So draw a box around "wad." Webster: "The cotton or silk obtained from the Syrian swallowwort, formerly cultivated in Egypt and imported to Europe." Oh. But read on: "A little mass, tuft, or bundle . . . a small, compact heap." Stet that one. I call this "the search for the mot juste," because when I was in the eighth grade Miss Bartholomew told us that Gustave Flaubert walked around in his garden for days on end searching in his head for *le mot juste*. Who could forget that? Flaubert seemed heroic. Certain kids considered him weird.

The editors

In the first draft, toward the end of the story, we have this passage (with your comments):

> Of course, that's not me.
>   [This is what I do: I take other lives and for short periods weave them through my own like threads of different but complementary colors.] **[rewrite]**
>   This is an interesting way to live; however, just as with talking with God, it keeps you from your responsibilities.

In later versions, this becomes:

> There it is: don't grow old with an unblemished heart. And don't **fear** death. If you never **fear** death, you'll always be free.

And then:

> There it is: don't grow old with an unblemished heart. And don't be afraid of death. Otherwise you'll never be free.

The line then remains untouched through several edits, until the very end of the process, when the author sends you a note to alter it into this final version:

> There it is: don't grow old with an unblemished heart. Be free. Don't be afraid of dying.

Drew

This passage followed the section in italics about the woman from the train: and so it has a great effect on how the reader interprets that section. To me, this is a perfect example of how a small and inexact prod from an editor can exact brilliance from a writer. The best kind of writer takes a vague comment like mine – "rewrite" – and gives you this, which is an entirely different animal. We resist, as a reader, the narrator's claim that "that's not me" – we don't want to be told that he does this, that he has woven this whole thread for our amusement: no, we want to be shaken by it, this love that wasn't, that couldn't be anymore than what it was. I felt, with that first draft, that he gave us something beautiful and then tried to take it away. These longings are why we live, why we read, never mind responsibilities. What we ended up with – "There it is: don't grow old with an unblemished heart" – doesn't try to say anything about whether or not the story is true, doesn't apologize or explain or any such thing. It is so much more powerful because it breaks from the scene and in some ways from the story, goes from what might be an admission of a significant affair and speaks directly to the people for whom it might matter – his wife, his four sons. No one can argue with this advice: don't grow old with an unblemished heart. If love presents itself to you, take it.

Of course, I should say that the line "That's not me" was intended to pick up the thread of an earlier line that followed an earlier section in italics. That section begins, *He stands in the kitchen in the evening, listening to her put their boy to bed; he is rinsing a plate in soft running water and there washes over him a sense of the extraordinary privilege of the moment . . .*

> Him: that's me. But it's also not. This scene never happened. . . . Yet it did happen, to me, in the fact of writing it; because to write something in fictional mode that is at least minimally convincing, paradoxically requires that one experience it, whereas this is, again paradoxically, *not* required when one writes convincingly in memoir: the simple announcement at the outset that *all this really happened* lifts the obligation of flawless accuracy. One must only master the voice of memory: *In the evenings I stood at the sink and listened to her put our boy to bed, she knew his books by heart, quoted them to him while she washed him and picked up his toys.* One does not have to experience or re-experience that moment. In that sentence, in fact, the rituals are out of order, one could not be experiencing it while writing it; but to the reader it is convincing enough, memory is enough: the past has proved itself; the present, contingent, like fiction, has not.

In that context, we are already set up to read these italicized passages differently. The whole piece washes back and forth between these poles. Some statements accumulate in poignancy because they're so nakedly true. The sentence that concludes the above section reads, for example: "Even now, at this late date, I want you to know me. This is overbearing, I realize." To say nothing of the lines that conclude the story.

The editors

At the galley stage, Passaro suggests the following last-minute changes:

- Change this sentence: *"She was not that tall and neither thin nor heavy, solid, rounded, voluptuous, with sturdy limbs."* to this> *She was not that tall and neither thin nor heavy; she was solid, rounded, sturdy, voluptuous.* And then add> *She was not one whose fire needed to be lit; it was burning already.*
- Add "after that," > *They might have seen each other once or twice again after that, but neither . . .*
- Change "Try not to fear death. Be free." to> Be free. Don't be afraid of dying.
- Cut "perhaps" in the following> Only self-consciousness and *perhaps* aesthetic and moral and cultural distaste.

Some of these are described (by Bill Pierce, AGNI's senior editor) as feeling like "retreats" and "the children of cold-feet re-readings." The implication here is that there are occasions where the editor has to be bolder than the author – and that there is a point at which one can edit too much. Editing, then, is not simply about pulling lines apart, letting things emerge, but at times, about restraint, preserving what is there. How much of the editor's role is to "hold the line"? And what specifically in these particular changes caused concerns that some of the story's original tone might be "damped down"?

Drew

It's interesting that you use the phrase "hold the line"; I think this happens with good collaborations, as it does with rewriting in general. A writer can get caught up in a particular zeal: cutting the proverbial ten percent, maybe, trying to get closer to the meat of things by cutting unnecessary descriptions, et cetera – in the right mood, an ungenerous one, maybe, we can go too far, can do, as Epstein put it, violence to our natural style. In going through these rounds and multiple drafts, you can sense where it starts to fall apart: the writer or editor is edging toward the door, unable to read the thing anymore, and begins to make rash or bad suggestions or decisions. It's the job of one or both of us to stop that from happening.

The editors

Passaro writes: "Your edits are outstanding . . . in recognizing, in a way I could never quite figure out, some fundamental cohesion problem in the stance of the piece" – and you describe the editing process for this story as a "true collaboration." We mentioned earlier the notion of restraint – that the editor's more dispassionate stance can preserve and protect from over-refining. Toni Morrison speaks of another thing, "imaginative recklessness," in the writer-editor relationship. Are the examples here of where you, as editor, have pushed Passaro, as writer, further in the story than he would have gone alone?

Passaro

Jen has mentioned the little prods that sometimes take one to unexpected places ("rewrite," for instance). In a different, more recent piece we worked on together, quite near the end of the process, when all was basically settled, a small question she asked – what did I mean by some vague allusion – caused me to think and discover what in fact I had meant; discover it for the first time. I put it in the piece and (for me) it altered the shape of the thing noticeably and fixed the lighting, as it were, brought in an extra lamp to get rid of the shadows. And really her query had been rather small and offhand. So I do not think of Jen ever "pushing" me as a writer where I "wouldn't have gone," but marking doorways I haven't sufficiently opened, rooms (of my own creation) that I haven't sufficiently explored or sufficiently shown the reader. *She* didn't know with the "rewrite" discussed above, or the simple query I mention here, where her prodding would take me; she didn't have an established idea of territory that needed to be covered. She felt the trapdoor under the carpet. Which requires a special sensitivity.

The editors

Robert Gottlieb said that "the editor's relationship to a book should be an invisible one," but Passaro refers, if lightly, to the different edits as the "Jen Variations," which seems to acknowledge that the editing process leaves a defined impression on the finished story. How much do you feel your own voice can be heard in the final version of the text?

Drew

I feel honored by that phrase, the "Jen Variations," even if it means I've gone against Robert Gottlieb. I would not say the editing changed Vince's story into anything other than what it already was, only perhaps a finer version of itself: but he would have to answer that.

Robert Gottlieb said that in order to edit well, one has to "surrender" to the work. Actually, he said, "The more you have surrendered to a book, the more jarring its errors appear." For me, this process works in the reverse. The more I surrender, the more I'm able to inhabit the story and work from there, so errors are less jarring to me – which is not to say that I don't see them. Tackling missteps in a story is a lot more fun if the story becomes as dear to you as though you had written it yourself. This is easy for me to do with Vince's work, less so with those pieces for which I am not so well suited. Bill Pierce has said that he tells the interns at *AGNI* that if they don't like a story or essay, they shouldn't edit it. (The "interns" are all graduate students in Boston University's creative writing program: such work is one of two possible requirements of a scholarship to the program, or at least it was for me when I was there.) This is probably good advice for interns (not to mention for productivity's sake: the amount of work done by just a few people in the *AGNI* offices is insane), but I tend to think it's a valuable exercise to work on something so far outside your style that it occasions dislike. I have certainly edited my share of prose I don't love – one doesn't always have a choice – and this points again to the importance of an editor's mutability, malleability, that shape-shifting into the voice of another: qualities you don't necessarily want anywhere outside the job of inhabiting someone else's prose. My practice, with work I don't love, is generally to put it off until the last possible moment, and then, groaning to the dog, read it and maybe write nasty things to amuse myself in the margins. But always, by the time I've finished inputting my changes from the paper copy and making notes to the writer, the story will have won me over to its side.

Back to the business of leaving too much of a mark: we've just finished editing another short story of Vince's for the spring 2016 issue of *AGNI* and I'm thinking of it in reference to your question because we spent the majority of our time discussing the beginning, which I felt was too soft, and detained us longer than necessary from an electric sentence that, to my mind, was the natural beginning of the piece. I told him I felt this way particularly because the ending was as close to perfect as any end-ing can be, and I wanted the same feel at the beginning. I know what Vince is capable of and I can't help but read with that in mind. There was this one particular creative use of "magic-lanterned" that I pounced on immediately. Vince responded,

> My writing is becoming, somewhat on purpose, denser and denser. I see no reason – except when I do – to be spare. I love, for instance (and am not of the school that what I love should be what I cut) the "magic-lanterned" verb. It makes me so happy every time I see it anew. This is something that it's hard to put up with, I realize. But I'm getting old and if I want to wear green slacks and loud jackets, or really, caftan and many rings in terms of my prose style, I'm generally going to. No reason not to now …

Which is maybe what he means by "Jen Variations" – too clean around the edges, which is actually a style of writing I don't particularly admire. My aim is always to find that place, different for every writer, where the writing really sings: Fitzgerald's "high white note," which Hunter Thompson talked a lot about, or, to use Hunter's words, that "high-water mark." All the time I knew him, Hunter was trying to get back to that place, something you just know when you hear it. The particular choices the writer makes in word and rhythm and punctuation and cast – all of it combines into something of magic. In Vince's case, in the above instance – that "no" – Vince was right, and his saying so, and my seeing it, allowed the piece to be what it is.

Passaro

Actually, that's *not* what I meant by "Jen Variations" – all I meant was for it to identify the versions that had been fixed by you. If any stylistic character can be assigned to them it's the sense of balance and strength you get reading sentences that work, in which nothing is wrong. I also find, reading the above, that I don't *really* believe in taking my language to the "caftan and many rings" stage of ornateness. But the longer you live with dedication inside the language, make it your professional and spiritual milieu, the more you enjoy its complexity. Funnily enough I just sent in the final signed-off galleys on that new story today, and again today I enjoyed, with spe-cial depth and pleasure, that "magic-lanterned" verb, though if it weren't late and costly I would have cut the last phrase of the sentence, which is off a bit rhyth-mically. It doesn't quite "breathe" correctly, by which I mean you, the reader, have your breath overextended somehow reading it. Language functions first as rhythm and sound; signification comes after. I would say that I have rarely, possibly never, encountered a professional editor who had problems with the meaning of sentences, words, the language, but I've suffered quite a few who didn't understand it as sound.

The editors

Passaro's own questions are informed and focused, and they make up a key part of the editing process, but he's experienced, technically as well as in broader creative terms. We wonder how far new writers in particular are actually equipped to ask the kind of questions that he puts forward, to understand that something isn't working, that there is a "fundamental cohesion problem" in the first place, even if they're unsure how to fix it. In your correspondence, Passaro writes, "Earlier today I was ... recollecting that the deeper I went into the language, the more I became the master of my own voice, the less able I was to see errors in printed text. I had been a proofreader for a living, and ultimately couldn't spell, couldn't catch typos, couldn't see the language at that level anymore." Clearly the editor's more detached, objective relationship to the story enables a different kind of clarity of vision, so [*to Vince*] what is the impact of working *without* this relationship?

Passaro

The creative writer in general suffers when he has a grammarian over his shoulder, or a style master, or any kind of extrinsic judge creating a racket. I suffered for years from this, in my twenties, and it took me a long time to find my own voice. The sound and meter of the language, the words themselves – the array of them, the availability of the one you want or need at a given moment – all these start out for the serious writer as machinery he or she must learn to master. And each in turn, as one approaches mastering it, gets internalized, ceases being a machine and becomes part of one's voice. Watch a musician, a pianist or guitarist, handling her instrument, managing all the keys, the strings, knowing where the fingers go next, maintaining the essential rhythm or meter or beat, left hand doing something utterly separate from the right hand ... It looks as natural as picking up a comb and gliding it through one's hair. This happens to you as a writer, if you write a lot, have a good ear and eye, and are edited well. The problem is you no longer notice some of the little errors. Or at least I don't: things I never would have let happen in my early years now happen: I'll misuse then for than, or type some incorrect version of their/they're/there, etc. I'm hearing and I'm typing as if to a voice and I don't even see the words in that way anymore. Of course, when I revise I do see such mistakes as those, but smaller ones get by. Language is such a public element, so constant a part of the atmosphere, that commonplaces and clichés slip in sometimes, no matter how good you are.

As for the first part of your question, as a teacher I know that working with younger talents, less experienced writers, is a different kind of task. You can't just say "cliché" or "ick" – you have to explain the thing a bit more. And with more explicit sympathy. They don't actually *know* that if you've heard it said that way your whole life, that means you SHOULD NOT say it that way again. Thus we are still burdened with "shocks" of red hair and people "padding" across the floor in their socks. No amount of vigilance will ever wipe it all out.

The editors

Thank you both very much for sharing the materials and thoughts with us.

3

"TO THE RAINFOREST ROOM: IN SEARCH OF AUTHENTICITY ON THREE CONTINENTS"

Orion Magazine, May 2011

Robin Hemley and Jennifer Sahn

At the core of the writer-editor collaboration between Hemley and Sahn lies that old chestnut of all writing: the distinction between truth and fiction. This binary, which has been deconstructed over and over in the last five to six decades, seems to keep haunting the work that has been named Creative Non-Fiction. For Hemley, the search for authenticity in a postmodern age where everything is a form of simulation and simulacra is nevertheless a must, because it reveals something about the way humans construct their world as stories.

For this reason, the case in front of you not only contains the published piece, the draft with edits, and a conversation, but also an email correspondence between the author and the editor. This exchange shows and highlights, in addition, the very "search" for authenticity, however lost a cause it may be. We can trace the construction of the story as such and deliberations on the content as much as we can see the editing for aesthetic reasons. In other words, Sahn as an editor does not just polish the piece on the basis of the final submitted manuscript but is involved at crucial stages to help the writer make certain decisions in relation to his research, his plans, the very character of the story, and structure. We see it is not a matter of making the author go down a certain road but being there, being available in the making of decisions. Sometimes it looks like Hemley is obsessed with some insignificant detail, which the editor could very well discard and tell the author not to worry about, but as any good editor knows, truth lies in such details one obsesses with, whether or not they end up in the final piece. Here editing is as much letting things brew for a while and being sensitive to the details that make or break a story.

It can be argued that this line from the text – "And so I present for your further confusion, if not edification, three rainforests" – sums up the truth of both writing and editing: there is a presentation that is as confusing as it is edifying, and as edifying as it may be confusing. Confusion is essential for truth. This is something that Sahn as an editor allows Hemley. As much as she pushes for clarity and precision, she allows for a dose of confusion, which is part and parcel of the writing and the editing processes.

"To the Rainforest Room: In Search of Authenticity on Three Continents"

Part one

The Allure of Easy Cheese

I'm in favor of Authenticity.

Maybe I should rephrase that.

I want everything in my life to be Authentic. I want to only eat Authentic Food and only have Authentic Experiences. When I travel, I want to travel authentically (hot air balloon, camel, steam railway). I want to meet Authentic People (family farmers, I think, are authentic; people you meet in the Polka Barn at the Iowa State Fair; members of lost tribes; chain-smoking hair dressers named Betty). I want to think Authentic Thoughts.

Actually, Authenticity baffles me. I first wrestled with the notion about ten years ago, when I was researching a book about a purported anthropological hoax. The Tasaday were "discovered" in 1971 in the southern Philippines leading an authentically Stone Age existence. They lived in isolation in the rainforest, had no metal or cloth except what had been given them by a local hunter, wore leaves, carried around stone axes, and, most authentically, lived in caves. The Western world fell in love with them and soon the Tasaday graced the cover of *National Geographic* and were the subject of countless breathless news accounts. No one could be more authentic than the Tasaday until 1986 when a freelance journalist from Switzerland hiked unannounced into their forty-five-thousand-acre reserve and was told through a translator that the famous Tasaday were nothing more than a group of farmers who had been coerced by greedy Philippine government officials into pretending to be cavemen.

My task was to unravel the mystery, to discover whether they were in fact a bald hoax or a modern-day version of our Pleistocene ancestors.

Before giving you the definitive answer, I'd like to interrupt this essay to bring you a word about Easy Cheese. If given a choice between the inauthentic (Easy Cheese!) and the authentic (cave-aged cheddar cheese from Cheddar, England, where it was invented a thousand years ago), I usually go for the authentic, unless of course I want Easy Cheese because sometimes that's what you want. This problem dates back to when I was in boarding school in 1974 and someone handed me a Triscuit (Original Flavor) topped with a vivid orange floret extruded from a can. What can I say? It tasted great. How can we hope to live authentically when we have been compromised by prior experience?

With that out of the way, we may proceed.

The Tasaday were neither Authentic Cavemen nor a hoax designed to fool the naïve public. They were, in fact, a poor band of forest dwellers whose ancestors had fled into the rainforest a hundred and fifty years earlier to escape a smallpox epidemic. They became Pseudo-Archaics (a term used by Claude Lévi-Strauss) and lived more or less unmolested until they were "discovered" and made poster children for authenticity, chewed around for a while in the imaginations of the fickle public, and then shat out onto authenticity's midden.

From time to time, I read sentiments like this: "For a few hours I lived in an alternative Africa, an Africa governed by a quiet glee and an innocent love of nature," and I think *your* quiet glee, buddy, *your* innocent love of nature. This sentence, by the way, is an authentic quote from an actual essay that appeared in a recent travel anthology. When I read it, I could get no further. I wondered what the writer thought he was doing experiencing his quiet glee in this alternative Africa? This sentimentalization of "Primitive Man" in harmony with nature seems akin to a hunter praising the pristine beauty of an elk head he's shot and mounted. The hunter can move but the elk can't. The authenticity tourist can and will depart the rainforest, leaving behind his tourist dollars and those irrepressibly authentic Africans twittering their gleeful songs on their kalimbas.

Nature declawed, stuffed, mounted. What then do we really want from the Authentic Destinations of our imaginations? And how do our perceptions of them differ from the Real Thing? When we think of an unspoiled place, how much do we need to strip away before we reach the desired level of authenticity? Strip Hawai'i of its inauthentic fauna and you're left mostly with bats.

The idea of an authentic place implies an unchanging one, which also makes it an impossibility.

My experience with the Tasaday has rendered me hyperaware of the aura of desperation and melancholy surrounding our common need for the Authentic, especially in regard to Place and People. Call it a sixth sense. If I were a superhero, this might be my special power, though it might also be my singular weakness, my kryptonite, which was, after all, the only thing that could kill Superman, a chunk of authenticity from a home planet he could barely remember. And no wonder – because neither he nor his home planet ever existed, except in our minds, where they continue to exist, and powerfully so.

And so I present for your further confusion, if not edification, three rainforests.

Part two

Lied Rainforest: Omaha, Nebraska

Overlooking the second-largest waterfall in Nebraska, I wish that I could meet the plumber of this fifty-foot marvel. I asked to meet the plumber, but my request, I guess, was not taken seriously, and so I've had to make do with the director of the Henry Doorly Zoo, Danny Morris. I suppose I had some doubts about visiting one of the world's largest indoor rainforests before I showed up (yes, there *are* others). So what if a Paradise Tanager settles on a branch here? It's still Omaha outside.

Why would anyone go to the bother of bringing the rainforest to Nebraska? It's my theory that Nebraska has developed a severe case of landscape envy.

Arbor Day: invented by a Nebraskan.

The only man-made national forest (Halsey National Forest) is in Nebraska.

The word *Nebraska* originates from an Oto Indian word meaning flat water.

People of my generation will remember with fondness the weekly TV show *Mutual of Omaha's Wild Kingdom*, starring Marlin Perkins, which ran from 1963 to 1985 and gave most Americans their first exposure to the conservation movement. Perkins might not have been from Nebraska (though he was a Midwesterner), but Mutual of Omaha, the show's proud sponsor, certainly was. It may be the most logical thing in the world that a state as mono-diverse as Nebraska would be infatuated with exotic flora and fauna. If the rainforest is the closest thing on Earth to the Garden of Eden, to which we always hold out hope for our eventual return, Nebraskans may simply be looking for a shortcut.

Perhaps that's what drove the Henry Doorly Zoo's former director, Lee Simmons, to bring the rainforest to Omaha. Simmons had traveled to many rainforests around the world, because a zoo such as Henry Doorly typically has a research component to its mission. In fact, in the actual disappearing rainforest of Madagascar, the zoo's staff and interns have discovered twenty-one previously unknown types of lemurs. One day, Simmons and others, including Danny Morris, taped two whiteboards together, set a perimeter, and started drawing things they'd like to have in their rainforest, including of course, the waterfall and a swinging bridge, de rigeur in any rainforest worth its mist.

Yes, it was planned, and yet planned to look unplanned, so that you might experience the rainforest as authentically as possible without the fear of lawsuits. In the jungle you hardly know what is in front of you and then you turn a corner and see a waterfall or monkeys in a tree, and Simmons wanted to replicate that sense so that you'll never be sure what you'll find. Yes, of course, it's simulated, but at the same time "accurate." Simmons sent his "tree artists" to the Costa Rican rainforest. "You could tell the difference when they got back," Morris says. "Their trees were a lot better."

Consequently, in the Lied Rainforest there are no surprises, and yet everything is surprising.

The white noise of water cascading from the waterfall is designed to mask the shrill voices of school children on their outings, as well as the many life-support systems required by the ninety or so subtropical species living within its 1.5 indoor acres. The eighty-foot tree in the center of the rainforest, cutting through its various levels, is made of polyurethane-reinforced concrete and is hollow, acting as a giant air duct, recirculating warm air from the ceiling of the eight-story-tall rainforest in the winter and venting it in the summer. The paths, a mixture of dirt and rock wool, which acts as a stabilizer, are roto-tilled. Walk up an artificial cliff to Danger Point, lean against the bamboo fence, and it wobbles to give the impression that it might give way at any minute. It won't. The bamboo is set on steel pegs. Gibbons, hidden in the foliage, hoot like kids. Scarlet macaws perch on palm logs beside the epoxy tree they've vandalized by chewing on its branches. Bats fly free in the building, and arapaima, grown from twelve inches, loll in their pools, resembling manatees.

All of it seems authentic in most respects but happily inauthentic in others. At six p.m. or so, when the zookeepers open the doors of the holding pens, the animals are there waiting patiently to go in for the night, clocking out, as it were, for supper. And no one's threatening to put a road through Lied Jungle. No one's mining for gold.

If we lost as much of the Lied Rainforest today as we will of the Amazon, the Lied would be gone by tomorrow. And that, of course, is a large part of the point.

"You can watch all *The National Geographic* and Discovery Channel you want," Morris says as we pause in front of a curtain fig with its labyrinth of roots that kids can climb through. "But you need to smell it, hear it, and feel the heat. When you put all that together, it makes a more lasting memory."

So what if this tree is in finely fitted segments that are keyed for easy removal and reassembly?

Morris frets in the age of Google that when everything is at our fingertips, nothing is actually touched, and the idea of the rainforest will become ever more remote to Nebraskans, as will the notion of anything authentic at all. He's noticed fewer field trips from the local schools (Morris himself started at the zoo over thirty years ago as a volunteer Explorer Scout). And the zoo staff has been talking recently of adding to the exhibits a Nebraska farm because so few Nebraskans have ever set foot on a real farm.

But doesn't the word *authentic* lose all meaning if applied too liberally? What is an authentic cup of decaffeinated coffee? An authentic polyester suit? What are the essential properties of an authentic family farm? An authentic family farm would seem to need – now I'm just speculating here – a family running it, rather than the well-meaning staff of a zoo. But that might just be me.

Morris and I walk effortlessly from the rainforest canopy to the riverbed, across three continents, passing pythons and other creatures we wouldn't likely see in the real rainforest and would actually hope to avoid. In this rainforest, the one thing you must not do is step off the path, but if you do step over the little rope you might just turn a corner and find something completely unexpected: an exit sign above a garage door big enough to drive a truck through.

We walk across a bat guano minefield through a smaller door next to the garage door and come upon a wide tunnel ringing the complex that seems straight out of a James Bond film. We've dropped into an entirely different realm now. The green exit sign, the garage door, and suddenly we're confronted by, what? No evil henchmen, no jungle drug lab, but wading pools, animal toys, a reverse-osmosis system, and doors that seem like metaphysical portals: one says "South America," another, "Malaysia."

It's here in these rooms, the holding pens for the animals, that the pretense of authenticity drops away. These rooms are the Lied Rainforest equivalent of the actor's dressing room and Morris enters respectfully, not wanting to encroach on the animals' down time, but also concerned that a Francois' Langur monkey might snatch my glasses. But the black monkey with its bulging abdomen regards me from its wildness, sees that I am of no importance to its world, and ignores me. Somehow, this moment of disregard strikes me as the most authentic of the day.

Part three

Arajuno Jungle Lodge: Ecuador

From a motorized dugout canoe on the Arajuno River, I see a mostly unbroken screen of foliage on either bank. A woman does laundry on one muddy bank while her naked toddler squats and plays. A couple of men run a machine in the water, dredging for gold. They can make up to $150 a day for about six grams. The river flows swiftly after several days of rain. A young man perched in the bow of the canoe, barefoot, wears a muddy T-shirt and shorts. He sees the same scene every day, and yet he seems mesmerized by it, as though the river is someone he has recently fallen hopelessly in love with, or perhaps he's daydreaming of his real beloved, waiting for the right spot where he can get a signal on his cell phone and text her. We pass a young man in the river fishing with a net. Ten years ago, before my companion in the canoe, Tom Larson, arrived, the man might have used dynamite to fish instead.

A wheelbarrow and two giant bamboo saplings that Tom is donating to the community of Mirador for erosion control lie in the canoe beside us. The canoe is the local taxi service, so we're also joined by a woman in her twenties who has been to the market. We pull up to a heavily forested bank – her stop. The woman, a Kichwa Indian like most of the locals here, gathers her belongings: a backpack, a large white sack, a live chicken she dangles by its ankles in front of her. Two children and another woman descend the fern-lined embankment to give her a hand, one child reaching into the canoe and grabbing the real treasure, a liter bottle of Coke.

We pull away again and soon pass a sight that seems nearly as incongruous as a garage door in the middle of a jungle. A billboard protected with a thatched roof sits in a mostly denuded spot on the sandy bank, a few desultory banana plants growing beside it. The billboard shows a local official nicknamed Ushito, smiling broadly and giving the thumbs-up sign. Behind the trees, barely out of sight and parallel to the river, bulldozers have recently carved out a muddy track that will someday be a road connecting indigenous communities that until now have been connected mainly by the river. The road is one of Ushito's campaign promises. And today is election day. In jungles like this, roads tend to lead to deforestation, formerly inaccessible tracts of old growth being too tempting for illegal loggers to ignore. But labeling them "illegal loggers" makes them sound foreign. For the most part they're locals, though the buyers they're selling to are not.

When we reach Mirador, invisible from the shore, the bamboo plants are unloaded with the help of the canoe's pilot and a couple of local boys. Tom, wearing his typical uniform – Arajuno Jungle Lodge cap, T-shirt, cargo pants, and sturdy rubber boots – instructs the men in Spanish what to do with the bamboo. The fastest growing bamboo in the world, these saplings, already seven feet tall, will grow into bamboo Godzillas in a short while.

In his mid-fifties and wearing wire rims, Tom speaks softly and has the bearing of someone who has nothing to prove but can easily prove anything he wants to prove, a lifetime of conservation knowledge always at the ready. When Larson first landed in the area in the late '90s and purchased the eighty-eight hectares that became Arajuno Jungle Lodge (sixty-five hectares of primary growth and the rest secondary), a multi-hued Paradise Tanager landed on a nearby branch, and Tom took this as an omen. This is paradise, he thought. A former U.S. National Park Service employee and Peace Corps official with a Masters from the University of Idaho in Environmental Interpretation, Tom Larson has been trying to balance the books between paradise and "progress" ever since. Over time, the Arajuno Jungle Lodge has transformed from a personal project to save a small swath of rainforest to an eco-lodge and now a nonprofit foundation dedicated to helping the locals earn a living while not destroying their birthright in the process.

Hence, the fast-growing bamboo that we've transported to Mirador, which not only controls erosion, but can be used as building material and its young shoots eaten. Several days before my arrival, some university students from Canada and the U.S. planted this same variety of bamboo on the western edge of Tom's eighty-eight hectares as a clearly visible boundary. "You'll probably be able to see it from satellites when it's grown," he says. His property abuts the Jatun Sacha Reserve, two thousand hectares of rainforest, where on any given day you can find people cutting down trees (and through which cuts yet another road, this one eight kilometers long, despite a toothless legal ruling saying it shouldn't be there). Tom's bamboo boundary is in part to let everyone know quite clearly that this is Tom's part of the forest. No one, no one local at least, would cut one of Tom's trees.

In the Make-of-it-What-You-Will Department: Tom Larson was born and raised in Omaha, Nebraska.

The center of Mirador is deserted when we arrive after a short hike along a muddy and tangled path. Tom thinks perhaps they've formed a *minga*, a work party, and are off helping someone build or paint something. A field of grass defines the place, surrounded by a sparse and unevenly spaced ring of huts, some thatched, some roofed with tin. Tom points out the local school. A couple times a year, a group of students from the U.S. comes to Mirador and adjacent Santa Barbara to do projects. This year the students painted the school. Tom leads me across the field to check on some solar panels languishing inside the small building. The residents used the panels, donated by a Spanish group several years ago, to power their cell phones, but the storage batteries have since died.

Along a muddy path cutting through waist-high grass, we hike back to the river and hitch a ride in a canoe across to Santa Barbara, where Tom wants to show me the results of the aquaculture project he initiated. Tom started the project because, well, the dynamite blasts were "scaring the shit" out of the ecotourists at his lodge. First rule of eco-tourism: keep dynamite blasts to a minimum.

What would it take to stop you from blasting the river? he asked the locals, and they said they'd stop dynamiting the fish out of the water if they had their own supply of fish. So Tom, in partnership with the Peace Corps and with help from local residents, built twelve fish ponds in four communities. The Arajuno Jungle Foundation and the Peace Corps supplied the first five hundred fingerlings of *cachama* (a native fish) and tilapia (the ubiquitous supermarket fish), plus two one-hundred-pound bags of fish food. After that, the communities were on their own. Tom sent out word that anyone caught fishing with dynamite would never get assistance of any kind from Arajuno. Dynamite fishing has been reduced by 90 percent, he claims. Additionally, the Arajuno Jungle Foundation (whose board is made up exclusively of Nebraskans) built the water system for the ponds with Peace Corps assistance and built another system to bring water to the village.

When you imagine a rainforest pool, it's almost certain that you do not imagine the fish ponds of Santa Barbara. These utilitarian holes have been gouged between huts with planks and muddy paths running between them, PVC and hoses snaking all around. One woman wears a T-shirt with the smiling face of Ushito! She scatters fish food on the still surface of her pond, and hundreds of two-month-old fingerlings swim to the surface – all tilapia, because cachama fingerlings cost more and are somewhat more difficult to care for. The people in Santa Barbara don't really seem to worry that cachama are indigenous (and thereby authentic) while the tilapia are not.

A couple of ponds look dirty. One that wouldn't hold water has been turned into a muddy volleyball court. Another is empty because its drunken owner fell out of his canoe and drowned.

In the center of the village, we sit with a few local men and chat. The most talkative is Jaime, who has a reputation as a drunk, but he's a good-natured drunk. He offers us *chonta*, the red palm fruit that appears once a year, about the size and shape of a roma tomato, and begins thanking Tom profusely for helping them with their fish and saying how proud he is of his community that they have stopped dynamiting the river. Jaime, who appears to have been swilling local hooch all afternoon, gives me the thumbs up sign. So do his companions. "Ushito!" they all yell in unison.

Back at the Arajuno Jungle Lodge, I'm enjoying an afternoon of quiet glee, swinging innocently in a hammock overlooking the river. Tom flips through a copy of *The New Yorker* I brought with me. He asks if I'd like to watch Pink Floyd's *The Wall* sometime this week? Sure. Why not? That's what I came to the rainforest for. The guide who brought me here from Quito, Jonathan, who grew up in Ecuador, but whose parents are American, lolls like me in a hammock.

"You hear that?" Tom says.

At first I don't, but then a faint whine separates itself from the birds and the river. "That's the sound of progress," he says.

Jonathan looks up, listens, says, "There's three of them at least," meaning three men working chainsaws somewhere in the forest.

"I used to stop what I was doing when I heard chainsaws and investigate," Tom says, bringing beers for all of us to two long picnic tables near the hammocks. "But why should I put my head on the chopping block when they're not going to do anything anyway?"

By "they," he means his neighbor and much bigger reserve, Jatun Sacha. By "chopping block," he means getting shot or blown up. He's found dynamite on the hood of his car before. Last year, a park guard was shot. A bullet grazed his head and when the police came to arrest the gunman, they found themselves in a standoff with the man's many armed supporters, most of them from Santa Barbara. The police turned and ran.

"I've gone to Jatun Sacha how many times?" Tom says. "If you go on any Thursday they're cutting down trees to sell at the bridge in San Pedro on Friday. I've told Alejandro, 'I don't even mention this to you anymore because you never do anything.' 'I don't do anything,' he says, 'because I can't do anything. The police don't do anything. The Ministry of the Environment doesn't do anything.'"

Alejandro, whom I've met, is the director of Jatun Sacha. With his shoulder-length hair, thin mustache, and tired eyes, he looks a bit like Don Quixote, which is probably not an entirely inappropriate comparison. Jatun Sacha sold the right of way for an oil pipeline to run through the reserve, and, in exchange, two community internet centers were constructed that allowed eighteen people to finish high school. He's doing the best he can. And by "the best he can," I mean he wins pyrrhic victories.

But if the notion of compromise isn't native to the rainforest, it has certainly taken hold here, kicking notions of authenticity from the nest. The tourist who clings desperately to the latter might console himself briefly with the idea that authenticity is a man-made concept (like Easy Cheese!). Before this was a rainforest, it was an ocean. Was it more authentic then? Notions of authenticity themselves are a kind of invasive species.

In any event, there's no way to keep commerce and its insatiable appetites at bay for long. A new international airport in Tena, fifteen minutes from Arajuno, is slated to open soon. Ushito's road will continue being built across the river but won't likely be finished before the next election. Once the road is complete, Tom contends, the forest will go.

"If I were to oppose that road," Tom says, "my name would be mud around here." Instead, he effects what positive change he can. His teeming fish ponds are stocked with giant cachama and handiaas well as native turtles he plans to restock in the river. And Arajuno bustles with projects for the community. A ceramics workshop. A workshop to train rainforest guides. A project to create medicinal plant gardens for indigenous communities. Even a French chef, training local women to cook meals using native plants for ecotourists at the various lodges in the region. My imagination takes flight and I envision pan-seared cachama with a chonta ragout. In this way, it's not just bellies that get fed, but fantasies, too, what we might call the Paradise of Cell Phone Coverage for the people of Santa Barbara, and what we might call the Paradise of Accessible Inaccessibility for the rest of us. A Paradise of Roadless Places with a way for us to enter. A Paradise of Contradictions.

Part four

The Greater Blue Mountains World Heritage Area

Rainforest and Scenic Railway: Katoomba, Australia. The Indiana Jones theme song welcomes me to my third and final rainforest, as I and about sixty other tourists, the largest contingent from China, crowd into a funicular that is open on all sides and covered with a green, cage-like mesh. To gain access to the Greater Blue Mountains World Heritage Area Rainforest and Scenic Railway, I purchased a ticket in the gift shop that entitled me to plunge, via the steepest funicular railway in the world, down to the forest floor and ride the Sceniscender, the steepest cable car in Australia, back up whenever I have seen enough to warrant the price of admission. And that will be whenever that invisible gauge in me that craves authenticity hits full.

I consider this a Bonus Rainforest, like an offer in which you buy two rainforests and get the third for free. Truthfully, I stumbled upon it. An hour ago, I was in suburban Australia, on a pleasant and tame street in the town of Katoomba, in a house overlooking a garden. But now I am caged and strapped into my seat on my way down the side of a mountain. In the spirit of adventure, I'm even wearing my Arajuno Jungle Lodge souvenir cap.

I'm visiting Katoomba on a retreat of sorts, the nature of which isn't important, except that it involves spending most of my time indoors, chatting amicably with a group of Australian writers, most of whom ask me daily if I've had the chance "to take a stroll down the path to the overlook!" Not one of them told me there was a rainforest there. You'd think this was something one ought to mention. Admittedly, one of them did describe it as "like the Grand Canyon but with trees."

Until now, Katoomba has seemed like another tourist town the likes of Park City, Utah, or Asheville, North Carolina, with sloping streets, pleasant houses, grocery stores, boutiques, and restaurants, and quaint architectural landmarks, in this case the grand Carrington Hotel, built in the late 1800s. To learn why it has the feel of a tourist town, go down Katoomba Street to Echo Point Road until you find yourself, almost without warning, facing an overlook as impressive as any in the world. Suburbia suddenly ends and a kind of prelapsarian fantasy begins as you gaze out upon seemingly endless miles of mountains, replete with rainforests and waterfalls and the giant stone pillars known as the Three Sisters. It is indeed like the Grand Canyon but with trees.

If someone had just uttered the magic word *rainforest*, I would have dropped everything to experience its majesty.

The exhibit, if we might refer to nature that way, can be found at the end of the funicular ride, where, upon disembarking, I find myself on a boardwalk surrounded by railings to protect the flora and fauna from me, as one sign admits. The forest floor is dominated by gum trees and a Chinese tour group with a harried, flag-waving guide who wants everyone to stay together. I want to get away from them, not because they're Chinese, but because they're human, and one of the reasons I go to the rainforest is to get away. I don't want to hear Chinese or English or French spoken. If in Ecuador, I want to hear the three low whistles of the undulated tinamou, a floor-dweller the size of a pheasant, answered by the longer and higher whistle of the little tinamou. If in Omaha, I want to hear the roar of a fifty-foot waterfall drown out hordes of schoolchildren. Here, I'd like at least a kookaburra with its almost stereotypical jungle call, the avian equivalent of *Ooh ee ooh ah, ting tang walla walla bing bang.*

I run down the boardwalk, pursued at a brisk pace by the Chinese. Signs along the path identify various plants, but I hardly have time to note them. I stop briefly at a Blueberry Ash, with its cluster of drooping white flowers, and also at a gray mound, a giant termite's nest, "home to a million termites or white ants." Ahead of me, a man speaks softly into his digital camera's microphone while jogging at a good clip and pointing the camera at the forest canopy. His efficiency and his lung capacity impress me, and I run after him just to see if I can keep up. His wife, also jogging, glances over her shoulder at me, seemingly alarmed, and I fall back. I would love to chat with them to ask why they're jogging as they film, how they think they'll remember this experience, but I'm too out of breath.

At a crossroads, one sign points to the Sceniscender, which will lift me away from this place and back to suburbia, but I'm not ready to be lifted. To the Rainforest Room, another sign proclaims, pointing in the opposite direction, and I think yes, "Tally ho! To the Rainforest Room!" I imagine a jungle glen, a stream, a twittering canopy in dappled light.

Ahead of me is an octagonal, open-sided building made of the kind of wood you'd build your back deck out of, with twelve benches and a trashcan in the middle. I sit down on one of the benches across from three young Australian women and one man, taking a breather.

"I think she's pretty," one of the women announces.

"No, not at all," the man beside her says.

"I think she's pretty in a European way," she says.

"No, not at all," he insists.

A sound separates from the conversation – faintly in the distance, not a chainsaw, but a plane, its insect whine claiming the empty space it glides across.

The Australians stand up to leave.

"I'd come back here," one of the women says.

"Not me," says the man. "No toilets."

I spot, a little way up the path, a flag waving frantically, drawing closer.

Half an hour later, the Sceniscender lifts me and about fifty other people back to the familiar world. We ride up and out of the jungle – past the Three Sisters, past a defunct roller coaster that was built over the gorge but never officially opened – and are delivered directly into the maw of the inevitable gift shop. Here, I can purchase any number of didgeridoos, placemats, and coffee mugs decorated with aboriginal art, stuffed toy wallabies, and outback hats. I resist.

Stepping out into the parking lot, I find myself thinking about how often our idea of what's real differs from what's actually there. And about how certain concepts persist in our consciousness long after they've disappeared. When the Dutch killed the last dodo on Mauritius in the 1600s, the idea of the dodo did not cease to exist. It became the poster bird for all creatures that are too stupid to save themselves. Still, any loss over time becomes more bearable. I can't authentically experience a dodo, but I can imagine it. I can Google a dodo, and in this sense get closer to a dodo than most people did who were alive when dodos still existed. And though dodos no longer walk the Earth, I saw a real dodo foot at the British Museum when I was eleven.

Maybe everything authentic eventually winds up an exhibit. Worse, maybe everything authentic eventually winds up depicted on a shot glass in a gift shop. Maybe the very idea of authenticity implies extinction. For the record, I'm *not* in favor of extinction. Here's one test: if you want to replicate it but can't, it's probably authentic. So maybe authenticity is something to be wished for, catalogued, but never owned. Something we can't quite pin down, but nevertheless yearn for. Something that, for a while anyway, can keep at bay the nightmare of a globe covered with polyurethane trees and inhabited by wild animals who clock out every evening.

The editing of "To the Rainforest Room: In Search of Authenticity on Three Continents"

The following text is the third draft submitted to Jennifer Sahn. The editor's input, which was handwritten and scanned, is marked in bold, including margin notes (marked as MN).

Part one

Rah Rah Authenticity [**MN: The Allure of Cheesz Whiz?**]

I'm in favor of Authenticity.
    [**Um?**] Let me rephrase that.
    I want everything in my life to be authentic. I want to [**only**] eat authentic food and only have authentic experiences. When I travel, I want to travel authentically (hot air balloon, camel, steam railway). I want to meet Authentic People (family farmers, I think, are authentic, people you meet in the Polka Barn at the Iowa State Fair, members of lost tribes, [**chain-smoking?**] hair dressers named Betty). I want to think Authentic Thoughts.
    Actually, Authenticity baffles me. I first wrestled with the notion about ten years ago when I ~~researched~~ **was researching** a book about a purported anthropological hoax in the Philippines. The Tasaday were "discovered" in 1971 in the Southern Philippines leading an authentically Stone Age existence. They lived in isolation in the rainforest, had no metal or cloth except what had been given them by a local hunter, wore leaves, carried around stone axes, and most authentically, lived in caves. The Western world fell in love with them and soon the Tasaday graced the cover of *The National Geographic* and were the subject of countless breathless news accounts. No one could be more Authentic than the Tasaday until 1986 when a freelance journalist from Switzerland hiked unannounced into their 45,000-acre rainforest reserve and was told through a translator that the famous Tasaday were nothing more than a group of farmers who had been coerced by greedy Philippine government officials into pretending to be cavemen.
    My task was to unravel the mystery, to discover whether they were in fact a bald hoax or our Pleistocene ancestors ~~brought back to life~~.

Before giving you the definitive answer, I'd like to interrupt this essay to bring you a word about Cheese Whiz. [But if Cheese Whiz offends, then by all means, skip the following paragraph, prop your eyes open with toothpicks à la *A Clockwork Orange*, and read Jean Baudrillard's treatise, *Simulacra et Simulation* (in the authentic French original, of course!).] [MN: I don't think an overly intellectual escape-hatch from Cheez Whiz-dom works here. Cut?]

If given a choice between the inauthentic (Cheese Whiz) and the authentic (Cave-aged cheddar cheese from Cheddar, England, where it was invented a thousand years ago), I usually go for the Authentic unless of course I want Cheez Whiz because, **let's face it,** sometimes that's what you want. ~~The~~ **This** problem ~~is that my taste buds were corrupted~~ **dates back to** when I ~~went to~~ **was in** boarding school in 1974 and someone handed me a Triscuit (original flavor) with a floret [swath? Blob?] of orange whiz on it. What can I say? It tasted great. How can we hope to never stray from Authenticity when we have been compromised by prior experience? [MN: Cheez Whiz comes in a jar. Easy Cheese comes in that can with the nozzle – and don't ask how I know this!]

With that out of the way, we may proceed.

The Tasaday were neither Authentic Cavemen nor were they a bald hoax designed to fool the naïve public. They were, in fact, a poor band of forest dwellers whose ancestors had fled into the rainforest a hundred and fifty years earlier to escape a smallpox epidemic. They became Pseudo-Archaics (a term used by Claude Lévi-Strauss) and lived more or less unmolested until they were discovered and made poster children for Authenticity, chewed on for a while by [in the imagination of?] the fickle public, and then shat out onto Authenticity's midden. [Archaeologists refer to the layered trash heaps they sift through as "middens." Authenticity's midden is the Tasaday rainforest, which has been whittled down somewhat since 1971, not so much by the gold miners and loggers who threatened the reserve in the early seventies, but by other tribespeople: the Manobo, the T'boli, and some lowlanders, all of them feeling the pressure to survive rather than preserve.] [MN: this feels muddy and unclear. Cut? Sharpen?]

From time to time, I read ~~published essays, contemporary essays, with~~ sentiments like this: "For a few hours I lived in an alternative Africa, an Africa governed by a quiet glee and an innocent love of nature," which sounds as though it was lifted from a Marlin Perkin's voice-over narration circa 1963 [MN: Are you stealing thunder from your more extended reference to Perkins and mutual of om. by using him here?]. When I read something like this I think, *your* quiet glee, *your* innocent love of nature. The idea of Authenticity is almost by definition static and so, impossible. [MN: The idea of an authentic place implies an unchanging one, which also makes it an impossibility?] When we think of an unspoiled place, how much do we need to strip away before we reach the desired level of Authenticity? Strip Hawai'i of its inauthentic fauna and you're left mostly with bats.

My ~~encounters~~ [experience?] with the Tasaday have created a hyper awareness [has rendered me hyperaware?] in me of the aura of desperation and melancholy surrounding our common need for the Authentic, especially in regard to ~~the~~

~~Authenticity of~~ Place and People. **[Call it a sixth sense?]** If I were a superhero, this might be my **special** power, though it might also be my **singular** weakness, my Kryptonite, which after all, was the only thing that could kill Superman, a chunk of Authenticity from a home planet he could barely remember. And no wonder because neither he nor his home planet ever existed, except in our minds, where they continue to exist and powerfully so.

And so I present for your further confusion if not edification, three rainforests. At the end of this essay, you will be given a short quiz.[1]

Part two

Lied Rainforest: Omaha, Nebraska

Overlooking the second-largest waterfall in Nebraska ~~in its fifty-foot majesty,~~ I wish that I could meet the plumber of this ~~rainforest, but imagine he or she is very busy~~ **fifty-foot marvel**. I asked to meet the plumber, but my request, I guess, was not taken seriously, and so I've had to make do with **director of** the Henry Doorly Zoo~~'s Director,~~ Danny Morris. I suppose I had some doubts **about visiting the world's largest indoor rainforest** before I showed up. So what if a Paradise Tanager settles on a branch here? It's still Omaha outside. Why go to the bother of bringing the rainforest to Nebraska? It's my theory that Nebraska~~, perhaps the most landscape-challenged state in the Union~~ has ~~for this reason~~ developed a severe case of Landscape Envy.

Arbor Day: invented by a Nebraskan.

The only man-made National Forest (Halsey National Forest) is in the panhandle of Nebraska.

In a flat **bald** land, the man with the one-foot sapling is King.

People of my generation will also **[?]** remember with fondness the weekly TV show, *Mutual of Omaha's Wild Kingdom*, starring Marlin Perkins, which ran from 1963–1985, and gave most Americans their first exposure to the conservation movement. Perkins might not have been from Nebraska (though he was a Midwesterner), but Mutual of Omaha, the show's proud sponsor, certainly was. Perhaps it's the most logical thing in the world that a state as mono-diverse as Nebraska would be Conservation HQ **[want to have love affairs with exotic landscapes?]**. It's the outsider who often sees the benefit of something he doesn't have. **On the other hand,** The rainforest as sacred Garden is our oldest mythic home, and we always hold out the possibility of our eventual return, no matter how unrealistic. Perhaps Nebraskans simply want to find a shortcut.

The Henry Doorly Zoo's former director, Lee Simmons, traveled to many rainforests around the world and wanted to bring the rainforest to Omaha. **[MN: was this his motivation, or research?]** So **one day** he and others including

---

1   In the email exchange, note the extent of discussion that went into the use of a quiz in the end, which was ultimately abandoned.

Danny Morris taped two whiteboards together, drew a perimeter, and started draw-ing things they'd like to have in their rainforest, including of course, the waterfall and a swinging bridge, *de rigeur* in any rainforest worth its mist. **[love this!]**

Yes, it was planned, and yet planned to look unplanned, so that you might experience the rainforest as authentically as possible without the possibility of lawsuits. In the jungle (~~the mighty jungle~~) you hardly know what is in front of you and then you turn a corner and see a waterfall or monkeys in a tree and Simmons wanted to replicate that sense so that you'd never be sure what you'll find. Yes, of course, it's romanticized **[simulated?]**, but at the same time "accurate." Simmons brought **[sent?]** his "tree artists" to the Costa Rican rainforest. "You could tell the difference when they got back," Morris says. "Their trees were a lot better."

Consequently, in the Lied Rainforest~~, the largest indoor rainforest in the world~~, there are no surprises, and at the same time, everything is surprising.

The white noise of water cascading from the waterfall is designed to mask the shrill voices of school children on their outings, as well as the many life-support systems ~~for~~ **required by** the 90 or so subtropical species of animals **living** within its 1.5 acres. The eighty-foot tree in the center of the rainforest, cutting through its various levels, is made of polyurethane-reinforced concrete and is hollow, acting as a giant ~~circulation~~ **air** duct, recirculating warm air from the ceiling of the eight-story tall rainforest in the winter and venting it in the summer. The paths are rototilled and mixed with rock wool, which looks like insulation, to make them more stable. Where there are no railings, the drop offs seem slight and harmless. Walk up an artificial cliff to Danger Point, lean against the bamboo fence on the cliff and it wobbles when you touch it to give the impression that it might give way at any minute. But it won't. The bamboo is set on steel pegs. Gibbons, hidden in the foliage, hoot like kids. Scarlet Macaws perch on palm logs beside the epoxy tree they've ruined **[defaced? vandalized?]** by chewing on its branches. Bats fly free in the building and arapaima, grown from 12 inches ~~and resembling manatees~~, loll in their pools **resembling manatees**.

All of it seems authentic in most respects but happily inauthentic in others. When **at 6pm or so** the zoo keepers open the doors of the holding pens ~~at 6pm or so~~, the animals are there waiting patiently to go in for the night, clocking out as it were, for supper. And no one's threatening to put a road through Lied Jungle. No one's mining for gold. If we lost as much of the Lied Rainforest today as we will of the Amazon, the Lied would be gone by tomorrow. And that, of course, is a large part of the point.

"You can watch all the National Geographic and Discovery Channel you want," Morris says as we pause in front of a curtain fig with its labyrinth of roots that kids can climb through. "But you need to smell it, hear it, and feel the heat. When you put all that together, it makes a more lasting memory."

So what if this tree is in finely fitted segments ~~and is~~ **that are** keyed for easy removal **[and reassembly?]**?

[Danny himself started as an Explorer Scout volunteer over thirty years ago, and the zoo still maintains at its core an active intern program, and sponsors field research on lemurs in the real disappearing rainforest of Madagascar. Twenty-one previously unknown types of lemurs have been discovered by the researchers, previously unknown to scientists because of the lemurs' nocturnal natures.] [**MN: Not essential. Cut?**]

And yet Danny [**Morris? Choose one**] frets in the age of Google, **that** when everything is at our fingertips, nothing is actually touched, and the idea of the rainforest ~~becomes~~ **will become** ever more remote to Nebraskans, **as will** the notion of anything authentic at all. He's noticed fewer field trips from the local schools. And the zoo staff has been talking recently of adding ~~among~~ **to** their exhibits a Nebraska farm because so few Nebraskans ~~in this farm state~~ have ever set foot on a real farm. [We know from the laws of thermodynamics that things tend to proceed from order to disorder, which doesn't mean that things stop existing but that they are rearranged, that one thing becomes a multiplicity of things. And if we ~~might~~ extend this law of physics for a moment to the realm of ideas, we might say that the idea of an authentic farm, like **the idea of** an authentic rainforest, becomes **more** complicated over time.] [**MN: Can you sharpen this at all?**]

Danny and I walk effortlessly from the rainforest canopy to the river bed, across three continents, passing pythons and other creatures we ~~likely~~ wouldn't **likely** see in the real rainforest and would [**actually?**] hope to avoid. In this rainforest, the one thing you must not do is step off the path, but if you do, ~~if you're so adventurous that you~~ step over the little rope ~~and leave the path~~, you might just turn a corner and [**next to? above?**] find something completely unexpected: an exit sign and a garage door big enough to drive a truck through.

We step past a threshold covered in bat guano and come upon a wide tunnel ringing the complex that would seem at home in [**seem straight out of?**] a James Bond film. [**MN: Is this the garage door threshold? Beyond the garage door? Somewhere else?**] The green exit sign, the garage door, and suddenly you're confronted by what? [**Something here, like: You're really off the map now.**] No evil henchmen, no jungle drug lab, but wading pools, animal toys, ~~animal carriers,~~ a reverse-osmosis system, ~~rooms~~ **doors** that seem like metaphysical portals. One door ~~reads~~ **says** South America, another Malaysia. It's here in these rooms, the holding pens for the animals, that the pretense of authenticity drops away. ~~Signs remind keepers that they must enter in pairs~~ — These rooms are the **Lied Rainforest** equivalent of the actor's dressing room and Danny enters respectfully, not wanting to encroach on the animals' down time ~~and~~ **but** also concerned that a Francois' Langur monkey might snatch my glasses. But the black monkey with its bulging abdomen regards me from its wildness, sees that I am of no importance to its world, and ignores me. Somehow, this moment of disregard strikes me as the most authentic of the day.

Part three

Arajuno Jungle Lodge, Ecuador

~~There's more than trees behind those trees on either side of the Arajuno River, but nothing visible~~ From ~~our~~ **a** motorized dugout canoe **on the Arajuno River**

~~through the~~ **I see a** mostly unbroken screen of foliage on either bank. A woman does laundry on one muddy bank while her naked toddler squats and plays. A couple of men run a machine in the water, dredging for gold. They can make up $150 a day for about six grams. The river flows swiftly after several days of rain ~~have made it swell~~. A young man perched in the bow of the canoe, barefoot, wears a muddy T-shirt and shorts. He sees this same scene every day, and yet he seems mesmerized by it as though the river is someone he has recently fallen hopelessly in love with, or perhaps he's daydreaming of his real beloved, waiting for the right spot where he can get a signal on his cell phone and text her. We pass a young man in the river fishing with a net. Ten years ago, before my companion in the canoe, Tom Larsen, arrived, the man might have used dynamite to fish ~~rather than a net~~ **instead**.

A wheelbarrow and two giant bamboo saplings that Tom Larsen is donating to the community of Mirador for erosion control lie in the canoe beside us. The canoe is the local taxi service so we're also bringing along **[transporting? joined by?]** a woman in her twenties who has been to the market. We pull up to a heavily forested bank – her stop. The woman, a Kichwa Indian like most of the locals here, gathers her belongings, a backpack, a large white sack, a live chicken she dangles in front of her. Two children and another woman come down the fern-lined embankment to give her a hand, one child reaching into the canoe and grabbing the real treasure, a liter bottle of Coke.

We pull away again and soon pass a sight that seems nearly as incongruous as a garage door in the middle of a jungle. A billboard protected with a thatched roof sits in a mostly denuded spot on the sandy banks, a few desultory banana plants growing beside it. [The billboard shows a local official nicknamed Ushito, smiling broadly and giving the thumbs-up sign. And somewhere out of sight, but just barely, there's a wide muddy track that will soon be a road. It's an old campaign promise to the people upriver who until now have used the river as their highway. But not for much longer. Today is election day.] **[MN: this needs just a little fleshing out. Where is the road? Has it been built? Did Ushito promise it?]**

When we reach ~~At~~ Mirador, invisible from the shore, the bamboo plants are unloaded with the help of the canoe's pilot and a couple of local boys. Tom, wearing his typical uniform ~~of~~ Arajuno Jungle Lodge cap, T-shirt, cargo pants, and sturdy rubber boots, instructs the men in Spanish what to do with the bamboo. In his mid-fifties and wearing wire rims, Tom speaks softly and has the bearing of someone who has nothing to prove but can **easily** prove anything he wants to prove ~~easily~~, a lifetime of conservation knowledge always at the ready. The fastest growing bamboo in the world, these saplings, already seven feet tall, will grow into bamboo Godzillas in a short while. Besides controlling erosion, the mature bamboo can be used as building material and the young shoots eaten. Several days before my arrival, some university volunteers from Canada and the U.S. planted the bamboo **[MN: the same bamboos?]** on the western edge of Tom's eighty-eight hectares of forest as a clearly visible boundary. "You'll probably be able to see it from satellites when it's grown," he says. His property **[MN: we need some basic background in his property, the Lodge, its mission, etc.]** abuts the larger Jatun Sacha Reserve,

2000 hectares of rainforest, where on any given day you can find people cutting down trees, where a road, eight kilometers long **[is this a different road from Ushito's?]**, cuts through despite the legal ruling saying it shouldn't be there. The bamboo boundary is in part to let everyone know quite clearly that this is Tom's part of the forest. No one, no one local at least, would cut one of Tom's trees.

In the Make-of-it-What-You-Will Department: Tom Larsen was born and bred **[raised?]** in Omaha, Nebraska.

When Larsen first landed here in the late '90s and purchased his eighty-eight hectares, sixty-five of primary growth and the rest secondary, a multi-hued Paradise Tanager landed on a nearby branch, and Tom took this as an omen. "This is paradise," he thought. ~~Fortunate for everyone involved that fate sent him a Paradise Tanager and not Ushito, giving him the big thumbs up sign. He might have thought twice though perhaps even Ushito with his campaign promises would not have dissuaded him. Tom has spent nearly his entire adult life balancing the books between paradise and progress.~~ [At nineteen, he lined up a job as a firefighter in the 1.7 million-acre Malheur National Forest in Oregon. A seasonal employee of the National Park Service for fifteen years, a wilderness ranger for eight, he signed up with the Peace Corps in 1988, was sent to Ecuador and distinguished himself on various projects as station manager in the Galapagos. Eventually, he returned to the States, working again for the Park Service before receiving a Masters Degree from the University of Idaho in Environmental Interpretation. Then in 1996, he rejoined the Peace Corps and became the Assistant Training Director. But it was not his dream to move to Washington, DC permanently and work for the Peace Corps, which is what he was offered in 2000. Instead of a DC condo, Tom decided to buy a piece of the rainforest and protect it.] **[MN: can you find a way to condense this by half?]**

The center of Mirador is deserted when we arrive after a short hike along a muddy and tangled path. Tom thinks perhaps they've formed a *minga*, a work party and are off helping someone build or paint something. A field of grass defines the place — ~~a bare field in the rainforest as noteworthy as a windbreak of oaks on a Nebraska farm~~ — surrounded by a sparse and unevenly spaced ring of huts, some thatched, some roofed with tin. Tom points out the local school. A couple of times a year, a group of students from the U.S. come to Mirador and **[nearby?]** Santa Barbara and do projects. This year the students painted the school. Tom leads me across the field — to check on the solar panels languishing inside the small building. Several years back, a group from Spain donated eight 100-watt solar panels to Mirador. The panels lasted two years and then the batteries died. It was a good deed but an odd one, an unsustainable project, ultimately as effective as supplying faucets and refrigerators to a community with no running water or electricity.

One day, Tom found the panels lying on the roof. **[MN: are the solar panels essential to this story? If so, can you condense this part as well?]** Black mold had formed so thick, the cells weren't even visible. New panels cost $1000 each — Tom purchased one from the community. Now they'd like to sell five of the remaining panels and keep the other two so they can charge their cell phones. There's no running water here and no electricity, but cell phones, *si*.

~~Through~~ **On** a muddy path cutting ~~across~~ **through** waist-high grass, we hike back to the river and hitch a ride in a canoe across to Santa Barbara, where Tom wants to show me the results of the Aquaculture project he initiated. Tom started the project because, well, the dynamite blasts were "scaring the shit" out of the ecotourists at his lodge. What would it take to stop you from blasting the river? he asked the locals and they said they'd stop dynamiting the fish out of the water if they had their own supply of fish. ~~The old we're-just-trying-to-feed ourselves-ploy~~.

Tom and the locals **[MN: does this mean Tom?]** built twelve fish ponds in four communities. The project supplied the first 500 fingerlings of Kachama (a native fish) and Tilapia (the ubiquitous supermarket fish), plus two one-hundred-pound bags of fish food. After that, the communities were on their own. And Tom sent out word that anyone caught fishing with dynamite would never work for him or get assistance of any kind **[MN: how many of "the locals" does he employ or assist?]**. Dynamite fishing has been reduced by 90%, he claims. Additionally, Tom and the Arajuno Jungle Foundation (whose board is made up exclusively of Nebraskans) built the water system for the ponds with the help of the Peace Corps and built another water system so the village could have water **[system to bring water to the village?]**.

When you imagine a rainforest pool, it's almost certain that you do not imagine the fish ponds of Santa Barbara. These utilitarian holes gouged between huts with planks and muddy paths **running** between them and PVC and hoses snaking through **all around** tell variations of the same story about life here. One woman wears a T-shirt with the smiling face of Ushito! She scatters fish food on the still surface of her pond and hundreds of two-month-old fingerlings come to the surface – all Tilapia because kachama fingerlings cost more and need more oxygen **[?]**. The people in Santa Barbara don't really seem to care that kachama are the more authentic **[indigenous?]** fish.

A couple of the ponds look dirty. ~~If anything is coming out of them, it's the Creature from the Black Lagoon, not dinner~~. One ~~pond~~ **that** wouldn't hold water and has been turned into a muddy volleyball court. Another is empty because its drunken owner fell out of his canoe and drowned ~~a few months back~~.

In the center of the village, we sit with a few ~~of the~~ local men and chat. The most talkative ~~of them~~ is Jaime who has a reputation as a drunk, but he's a good-natured drunk ~~at least~~. He offers us *chonta*, the red fruit of a palm that appears once a year, about the size and shape of a roma tomato, and ~~launches into a speech~~ **begins** thanking Tom profusely for helping them with their fish and saying how proud he is of his community that they have stopped dynamiting the river. Jaime takes another pull of the local hooch he's been swilling all afternoon and gives me the thumbs up sign. So do his companions. "Ushito!" they all yell in unison. ~~Grateful as he might be to Tom,~~ **It** is after all election day ~~and Tom doesn't have a nickname (that he's sharing) or an optimistic hand gesture to make everyone feel that things are just going to keep getting better and better~~.

Back at the Arajuno Jungle Lodge, I'm enjoying an afternoon of quiet glee swinging innocently in a hammock ~~by a railing~~ overlooking the river. Tom is ~~at the dining table,~~ flipping through a copy of *The New Yorker* I brought with me. He asks me if I'd like to see **[watch?]** Pink Floyd's The Wall ~~concert~~ sometime this week? Sure. Why not? That's what I came to the rainforest for. ~~The Wall.~~ The guide who brought me here from Quito, Jonathan, who grew up in Ecuador, but whose parents are Americans, lolls like me in a hammock.

"You hear that?" Tom says.

At first I don't, but then a faint whine separates itself from the birds and the river. "That's the sound of progress," he says.

Jonathan, looks up, listens, says, "There's three of them at least," meaning three men working chainsaws somewhere in the forest.

"I used to stop what I was doing when I heard chainsaws, and investigate," Tom says, bringing beers for all of us to ~~the~~ two long picnic tables near the hammocks. "But why should I put my head on the chopping block when they're not going to do anything anyway?"

By "they," he means his neighbor and much bigger reserve, Jatun Sacha. By chopping block, he means getting shot or blown up. He's found dynamite on the hood of his car before. Last year, a park guard was shot. A bullet grazed his head and when the police came to arrest the man, they found themselves in an armed standoff with practically the entire community **[MN: which? where?]**. They turned and ran.

"I've gone to Jatun Sacha how many times," Tom says. "If you go on any Thursday they're cutting down trees to sell at the bridge in San Pedro on Friday. I've told Alejandro, I don't even mention this to you any more because you never do anything. I don't do anything he says because I can't do anything. The police don't do anything. The Ministry of the Environment doesn't do anything."

Alejandro, whom I've met, is the director of Jatun Sacha. With his shoulder-length hair, thin mustache, and tired eyes, he looks a bit like Don Quixote, which is probably not ~~too~~ **an entirely** inappropriate ~~a~~ comparison. Jatun Sacha sold the right of way for an oil pipeline to run through the reserve ~~(was there much choice?)~~ and in return, the **[oil?]** company **[MN: do you know the name?]** constructed two community internet centers which allowed 18 people to finish high school. He's doing the best he can. And by "the best he can," I mean he wins pyrrhic victories.

But if Ideas and Attitudes were separate species, then the natural habitat of the Compromise would be the rainforest **[MN: I like the idea of this sentence but can't quite do the math.]**. There is a road **[MN: is this Ushito's road?]** being built across the river, but we can't see it from our hammocks. "If I were to oppose that road," Tom says, "my name would be mud around here." Instead, he effects what positive change he can. His teeming fish ponds are stocked with giant *kachama* and *handia* as well as native turtles he plans to restock in the river. And Arajuno bustles with projects for the community. A ceramics workshop. A workshop to train rainforest guides. Even a French chef, training local women to cook meals using native plants for ecotourists at the various lodges in the region. Not simple *chonta,* as we sampled it in Santa Barbara, but perhaps broiled *kachama* with a *chonta* ragout? In this manner, more than bellies get fed, but fantasies too, what we might call the Paradise of Cell Phone Coverage for the people of Santa Barbara, and what we might call the Paradise of Accessible Inaccessibility for the rest of us. A Paradise of Roadless Places with a way for us to enter. A Paradise of contradictions. ~~But the searcher for Authenticity must get used to contradictions. They're part of the territory, a not uncommon species.~~ [MN: this feels to me like a really strong end to the Arajuno section. What follows, mostly seems to draw things out. Unnecessarily. Can you imagine parting with the next page and a half?]

The next day, Tom takes me on a tour of the old growth part of the rainforest. "Mona loves to take this walk," he says. "She just eats the entire way." Mona, an endangered Wooly Monkey, is two years old and was adopted by Tom near the Peruvian border after her mother was shot. She weighs about fifteen pounds, has a black head and a bushy tail. Tom picks her up by that tail now, dangles her for a bit, then drops her, while she acts completely unfazed, inspecting the path. Mona has a love/hate relationship with many of Arajuno's guests (by which I mean, me and Jonathan). She threw Jonathan's cell phone under the lodge yesterday. Mona is at times a little too Authentic. I wish she'd tone down the monkey act. If she were animatronic, I might not mind so much.

Soon, she's in the trees above us again while Tom takes out his Blackberry to check the signal. He can only get a signal from the top of the ridge that forms a kind of natural boundary between the more developed part of his property with its fish and turtle ponds, and the dip into the old growth forest. Efficiently, he retrieves his email and then we begin the steep dip along a path of tree roots and mud – Tom bushwhacks part of the trail with his machete and when we reach the old growth, he points out what looks like a fallen tree snaking across the forest floor. He follows it and I follow him and his machete until he stops and tells me to look up. The fallen tree is actually a buttress root and it belongs to an enormous tree, one of a pair Tom calls the Twin Towers. As I stand there admiring the Authentic Rainforest, Mona makes a point – perhaps the point that this is a real place and not just in my head – by nearly killing me when she sends a huge branch crashing onto my hand. "She meant to do that, you know," Tom says.

We hike along a wide, rock-strewn stream for a while and then we have to make a decision. "We can keep following the stream," Tom says, "or do a fairly strenuous climb where there's another spectacular tree."

"I'll opt for the less strenuous," I tell him and we start downstream, but then I change my mind. I am, after all in search of Authenticity. So we clamber up a narrow and slippery path with drop offs that might well finish what Mona started. Along the way, he shows me a *pambil* tree with stilt roots, maybe a genetic holdover, he says, from when this area was underwater. Something as primal as the rainforest was once underwater? It was once more Authentic than it is now? It's odd to see things here that I've only seen before now in supermarkets or in the living rooms of elderly relatives: Christmas cacti and a monster philodendron. There are certain plants that seem too . . . civilized to actually warrant a natural habitat. Seeing things familiar grown enormous makes me feel as though I'm in one of Henri Rousseaus paintings, the postal clerk who painted jungles of Parisian houseplants patrolled by tigers.

Tom picks something off the ground. It's an ant. A Lemon ant, he calls it. When you bite, it sends out a poison, but the poison is harmless to us. It tastes pleasant. He hands it to me and without hesitation I put it in my mouth and bite. Indeed, I can almost forget that this ant isn't in fact an authentic lemon.

Part four

The Greater Blue Mountains World Heritage Area Rainforest and Scenic Railway: Katoomba, Australia

The Indiana Jones theme song welcomes me to ~~this~~ **[my third and final?]** rainforest as I and about sixty other tourists, the largest contingent from China, descend a narrow shaft of the mountain **[?]** in roller coaster-sized cars, open on the sides and covered with a green cage-like mesh on top. To ~~get~~ **[gain access?]** to this rainforest in the Blue Mountains, I purchased a ticket in the gift shop that entitled me to take the Scenic Railway, the steepest funicular railway in the world, **down** to the forest floor, and the Sceniscender, the steepest cable car in Australia, back up whenever ~~it is~~ I have seen enough scenes to seem worth **[warrant?]** the price of admission. And that will be whenever that invisible gauge in me that needs **[craves?]** ~~the Paradise of~~ Authenticity hits full.

I consider this a Bonus Rainforest, like an offer in which you buy two rainforests and get the third for free. Truthfully, I stumbled upon it. An hour ago, I was in Australian suburbia **[Suburban Australia?]**, on a pleasant and tame street in the town of Katoomba, in a house overlooking a garden. ~~, and~~ **But** now here I am, **caged and strapped into my seat,** on my way down the mountain to the Actual Rainforest. ~~caged and strapped into my seat, but full of~~ **In** the spirit of adventure. I'm even wearing my Arajuno Jungle Lodge souvenir cap.

~~I'm in~~ **I was visiting** Katoomba ~~for a week~~ on a retreat of sorts, the nature of which isn't important, except that it involve~~s~~**d** spending most of my time indoors, chatting amicably with a group of Australian writers, most of whom ~~have~~ asked me daily if I'~~ve~~**d** had the chance "to take a stroll down the path to the overlook!" Not one of them told me there was a rainforest ~~t~~here. You'd think ~~that~~ **this** was something one ought to mention. Admittedly, one of them described it as "like the Grand Canyon but with trees." Still, that wasn't quite enough to get me off my duff until today, my last in Katoomba. If someone had just uttered the magic word, "rainforest," I would have dropped everything to experience its majesty.

~~But~~ **The** feeling of being in a cage only increases when I step off the funicular and find myself in a cage. Not exactly a cage. The exhibit, if we might refer to Nature **[MN: love this!]** that way, is designed like an ant farm in which the creatures make their little tunnels enclosed in a transparent terrarium. In this case, the tunnels have been pre-burrowed through the rainforest. **[MN: this description needs to be crispier. I can't quite picture it.]** I'm on a circuit of several kilometers of boardwalk surrounded by railings and netting to protect the flora and fauna from us, as one of the signs admits. The bottom of the forest floor is dominated by a Chinese tour group with a harried, flag-waving guide who wants everyone to stay together. I want to get away from them, not because they're Chinese but because they're human, and one of the reasons I go to the rainforest is to get away. I don't want to hear Chinese or English or French spoken. If in Ecuador, I want to hear the three low whistles of the Undulated Tinamou, a floor-dweller the size of a pheasant, answered by the longer and higher whistle of the Little Tinamou. If in Omaha, I want to hear the roar of a fifty-foot waterfall drown out hordes of schoolchildren. Here, I'd like at least a Kookaburra with its almost stereotypical jungle call, the bird **[avian?]** equivalent of Alvin and The Chipmunks singing "Ooh ee ooh ah ah, ting tang walla walla bing bang."

I run down the boardwalk, pursued at a brisk pace, by the Chinese. Signs along the path identify various plants, but I hardly have time to note them. I stop briefly at a Blueberry Ash with its clusters of drooping white flowers and also at a giant termite's nest, "home to a million termites or white ants." Ahead of me, a man speaks softly into his digital camera's microphone while jogging at a good clip and pointing the camera at the forest canopy. His efficiency and his lung capacity impress me and I run after him **[just?]** to see if I can keep up. His wife, also jogging, glances over her shoulder at me, seemingly alarmed, and I fall back. I would love to interview them **[for this story?]**, to ask them why they're jogging as they film, how they think they'll remember this experience. But I'm **[too?]** out of breath.

At a crossroads, one sign points to the Sceniscender, which will lift me away from this place **[and back to suburbia?]**, but I am not ready to be lifted. "To the Rainforest Room," another sign proclaims, pointing in the opposite direction, and I think yes, "Tally ho! To the Rainforest Room." ~~That's where I'll go, my place of refuge~~. I imagine a jungle glen, a stream, a twittering canopy in dappled light. I imagine innocence and quiet glee **[MN: used on p. 13]**. An alternative Australia, Africa, South America, Europe, Asia, North America. Thumbs up. Ushito!

Ahead of me is an octagonal open-sided building made of the kind of wood you'd build your back deck out of, with twelve benches and a trash can in the middle. I sit down on one of the front benches across from three young Australian women and one man, taking a breather.

"I think she's pretty," one of the women announces.

"No, not at all," the man beside her says.

"I think she's pretty in a European way," she says.

"No, not all," he insists.

They stand up to leave.

"I'd come back here," another woman says.

"Not me," says the man. "No toilets." **[MN: end here?]**

[Undoubtedly, somewhere in Australia, there are Nebraskans at this very moment working their magic on behalf of the landscape. This is what Nebraskans do, I gather, much like Israelis making the desert green. But if Nebraskans lurk nearby, I've so far managed not to spot them.] **[MN: this attempt to connect Nebraska doesn't quite succeed, but it could.]** As the first group leaves, another couple approaches the room but turns around when they discover it's nothing much at all.

Slowly, the human sounds fade and I start to hear birds sitting in their trees outside of the rainforest room.

A sound separates from the rest, not a chainsaw, but a plane, its low insect hum claiming the empty space it glides across. A little up the path, I spot a flag waving frantically, drawing closer.

Part five [MN: this needs to be funnier]

A Brief Questionnaire: How Authentic Are You?

Unlike most quizzes, you're the only one who can decide which answers are correct.

1. Which is the most authentic activity Rainforest People can engage in?

    A. Mining for gold
    B. Cutting down trees
    C. Fishing with dynamite
    D. Living in harmony with nature

2. Of the three rainforests, I visited, which is the most Authentic?

    A. The Lied Rainforest
    B. The Arajuno Rainforest
    C. The Greater Blue Mountains World Heritage Rainforest and Scenic Railway
    D. All of the above
    E. None of the above
    F. All of the above and none of the above

3. Ushito's grandfather is being chased by something through the rainforest. What is it?

    A. A bulldozer
    B. A photographer
    C. A missionary
    D. A house cat gone feral named Scamper Jack

4. If a road is built in the rainforest, this will inevitably lead to (mark all applicable answers):

    A. Deforestation
    B. Access to education and medical services
    C. Ushito's re-election
    D. Nebraska

5.   When we look for Authenticity we're really looking for:

    A. a pipe dream (though a pipe made out of sustainable bamboo)

    B. Inner Peace, Sanctuary

    C. Hope

    D. A photo op

From pitch to publication
Correspondence between Robin Hemley and Jennifer Sahn

The following are selected excerpts from the correspondence between Hemley and Sahn, from the initial pitch in April 2009 to the final stages of the editing process in 2011, including a note on Hemley's Pushcart Prize win in 2012. The correspondence shows a complex process of writing a creative non-fiction story, the effort and patience, and a commitment to a theme.

The pitch

Dear Jennifer Sahn,

My friend Suzanne Paola suggested that I get in touch with you about possibly writing a piece for *Orion*. My name is Robin Hemley, and I'm the author of eight books of nonfiction and fiction, including the forthcoming DO OVER! from Little, Brown (May 11, 2009). I've received a Guggenheim Fellowship and many other awards for my writing including two Pushcart Prizes, The Nelson Algren Award from *The Chicago Tribune*, and the Independent Press Book Award for Nonfiction, to name a few. I've published extensively in such places as *The Wall Street Journal*, *New York Magazine*, *The Chicago Tribune*, *Far Eastern Economic Review*, and I write a column for *McSweeney's* Internet Tendency, "Dispatches from Manila."

    I'm traveling soon to the Arajuno Jungle Lodge in Ecuador, run by the Arajuno Foundation, a place in the rainforest that combines eco-tourism with projects intended to help local indigenous communities as well as reintroducing endangered species into the wild. The AJL property consists of 65 hectares (161 acres) of primary forest [jungle], 20 hectares (50 acres) of secondary forest, and a three-hectare (7.5 acres) agro-forestry system.

    In any case, I've written a proposal that I'd like to share with you if you're interested. The piece I propose to write is only partly about Arajuno, but also about Omaha, Nebraska and Dekorah, Iowa and the connections between these places.

    If you'd like to see the proposal, I'd be happy to send it your way. You can also see examples of recent work on my website Robinhemley.com

    Thanks much for your time.

Sincerely, Robin Hemley

The proposal: one place is the same as another

I'm going down to Ecuador to spend a few days at the Arajuno Jungle Lodge, part of the Arajuno Jungle Foundation, an organization dedicated to preserving the rainforest and helping indigenous people with sustainable eco-tourist projects. One of the main organizers of the lodge is a man named John Van Gundy, a graduate of the Nonfiction Writing Program at the University of Iowa, where I teach. The Arajuno Foundation is busy on many fronts – the great grandson of Charles Darwin was a recent visitor, and the Lodge is constantly involved in monitoring endangered species and reintroducing them into the rain forest. Besides this, they engage in a number of creative projects designed to help the local indigenous population, including an intensive cooking workshop, led by a well-known French chef, to train indigenous women to cook healthy meals for the ecotourists who are more and more a part of the landscape all over the region. There's also training in basket weaving and the kinds of crafts that were known to the ancestors of the locals but have become increasingly forgotten.

I know something about the rainforest and notions of "primitivity" and "Authenticity," having published a well-received book in 2003 with Farrar, Straus, and Giroux, on a purported anthropological hoax in the Philippine rainforest, INVENTED EDEN.

My goal is to pair my trip to Ecuador with a trip to Nebraska. Why Nebraska? The owner/operator of AJL is a native Nebraskan, as are all of the founding Board members of AJL. When we think rainforest, we naturally think "Nebraska," right? The state tops my list of most boring to drive through and least likely to inspire save-the-earth type projects. Or because it IS so mono-diverse, it's exactly the place where the bio revolution starts: After all, the Henry Doorly Zoo in Omaha boasts the best enclosed rainforest exhibit (approximately 20 acres on three levels), Arbor Day was started in Nebraska and Arbor Lodge is located in Nebraska City, Nebraska. Finally, the only man-made National Forest (Halsey National Forest) is in the panhandle of Nebraska.

My own Midwestern state, Iowa, recently tried to rival Nebraska in the man-made rainforest department when they tried to build a 24-hectare indoor rainforest in the strip mall oasis of Coralville, Iowa (the project fell through, but not before Congress earmarked 24 million for the project).

As Michael Pollan showed us in OMNIVORES DILEMMA, the family farm in Iowa is about as endangered as the rainforest in Ecuador. My last stop in my journey would be another Midwestern destination: Seed Savers in Dekorah, Iowa, a farm that is the Midwestern equivalent of Arajuno Jungle Lodge. People from around the U.S. send heirloom seeds to this farm, which grow them for the same reason that AJL sends baby turtles back into the jungle rivers, to preserve the dying notion that one place is not necessarily the same as another.

Finally, I'm always quick to criticize people for "exoticizing," but on the other hand, it's perhaps the very romanticizing of the rain forest and the Iowa farm by people who don't live there and will never see either one, but who still need to imagine they exist, that will save them.

Note: This proposal was shortly amended.

22 April 2009
Hi again, Jennifer,

I just wanted to say that the last paragraph of my proposal in some ways should be the first, the idea that it's our imaginings of an ideal rain forest or an ideal Iowa farm, especially farms and rain forests that we have somehow exoticized, that fuels our desire to conserve and revive them. These real places are given life by our imaginations and in turn without the knowledge that such places exist and thrive, our imaginations might atrophy as well.

All the best, Robin

28 September 2009
Dear Robin,

I like the setup of putting three places in some kind of narrative conversation with each other. And I like that the piece seems to have some kind of tourism angle, but that the angle is in part a critical one. What I like most of all is that it seems as if a triangulation between these three places should drop you, the narrator, in ideal territory to make some kind of statement or conjecture about authenticity, which is a supremely important and oft-undervalued quality in modern society.

I think, however, that I am reading between the lines of your pitch. I didn't get a terribly strong sense of what kind of story was being framed, or what kind of connections you would be likely to draw between these places. That's understandable. This kind of piece can be pretty hard to pitch, and equally hard to commission, because success lies almost entirely in the execution. But if we are talking about a literary sort of narrative, grounded in scene and setting, with a solid "think piece" center, then I am pretty interested.

Do let me know where you are with this idea, and if what I've said here seems congruent with your own thinking.

All the best, Jennifer

3 October 2009
Dear Jennifer,

A few further thoughts on my "One Place" idea. One thing that strikes me as especially intriguing is how complicated the notion of authenticity is (something that has long intrigued me) and how different notions of authenticity often compete with one another or are at odds with the wishes of locals/natives. At Arajuno when I visited for instance, hundreds of trees had been cut down and a road bulldozed almost overnight across the river from the Arajuno Jungle Lodge. Tom Larsen, owner of the lodge, was appalled in a resigned way. Traditionally, the Arajuno River has been the highway for the people there, but the new road will connect a couple of remote villages (that Tom has been helping with aqua culture projects) to the larger world of commerce. Tom is also repopulating the river with native turtles and has helped the Arajunos to create fish ponds with the fingerlings of a variety of local fish. But the locals prefer Tilapia because Tilapia reproduce faster, take less care, and cost less to buy.

That's the first stop on my authenticity tour . . .

In preparation for my trip to Seed Savers, I've been looking at their website and see that they are embroiled in a battle over authenticity and what it means as well. The co-founder of Seed Savers (founded in 1975) was fired by the Board and has written at least a couple of open letters to all the members of Seed Savers deriding the "loss of vision" of the Board, for among other things, supplying heirloom seeds to the Svalbard Seed Vault in Norway, dubbed by the media as "The Doomsday Vault." As one member writes, "Kent points out that SSE's deposit of seeds in the Svalbard is the only deposit from a private company. He points out concerns over any country being able to request seeds from Seed Savers. Because of the signed agreement and the linked FAO Treaty, Seed Savers cannot deny a request for seed. His main concern is the ability for companies to genetically alter those seeds and then patent those derivatives. My question is: **Why is Seed Savers depositing seed in a seed vault whose main goal is to breed new varieties?** The summer harvest edition from Seed Savers on page 30 goes into great detail on this topic. I always was under the impression that Seed Saver's main goal was to recover and maintain heirloom varieties. These varieties already show great diversity. Seed Saver members certainly breed new varieties but this doesn't seem to be the main focus of the organization. This coupled with questions over patents does indeed raise concerns." I'd like to spend a couple of days up at Seed Savers and also track down Kent Whealy and get his version of the controversy in his words . . .

Last, I still want to visit the biosphere in Omaha that has one of the largest indoor rainforests in the world. The project is starting crystallize for me, and I hope you can see in the above two examples the possibilities here. My question to you is whether this seems to you as something you'd like to sponsor, if you will. My track record is excellent, I think. I've written articles and essays for many well-known publications, have been widely anthologized, and won a Guggenheim for my work last year. If you would like to chat further about this, perhaps we could find a time to talk on the phone? Thanks much for your consideration.

All the best, Robin

9 October 2009
Yes, I would absolutely like to talk further about this and try to get something off the ground. Maybe we can make a phone date for next week?

Jennifer

13 October 2009
Hi again, Jennifer,

If we could chat sometime this week or next, that would be great. I'm tentatively planning to drive up to Seed Savers in Decorah, Iowa on October 23rd and then to the Henry Doorly Zoo (home of the "best" enclosed rainforest in the world) in Omaha on November 16th. In Omaha, I'll be meeting with one of the Board of directors of Arajuno Jungle Foundation, which I visited in April. After the 16th,

I believe I'll have enough to write my piece on authenticity – I'm really interested in the ways our notions of authenticity change and are compromised by "Real Environmental Politik" (to coin a phrase), though perhaps realpolitik is perhaps too pejorative a term. I'm not interested so much in condemning compromise as I am in exploring it. Hope that interests you as well.

All the best, Robin

24 October 2009
Hi Jennifer,

I just wanted to let you know that I went up to Seed Savers yesterday and had a great visit. Not only did I speak with the new Executive Director but also with the co-founder, Diane Ott Whealy. My conversation with her was especially fruitful (no pun intended), and we circled around the controversy with her ex-husband Kent. We talked a lot about authenticity, honesty, and purity. I'm quite excited about the piece and will be traveling to the Henry Doorly Zoo in Omaha in mid-November. I hope I'll be able to give you the essay even before the end of the year …

Likewise, I'd fallen a little behind in my reading of Orion of late, and I just wanted to tell you how much I enjoyed all the pieces in the latest issue. It was great seeing Lia Purpura's piece – she's a good friend and in fact I'm giving a reading next month at her college. I also loved that piece about growing up hard in Montana and the walking pieces. Everything was strong. Those were just my favorites.

All the best, Robin

23 December 2009
Hi Jennifer,

I hope all's well. I just wanted to update you on my piece and ask if I might have a small extension? I'd like to change the piece just a bit, I think, as a result of a recent trip to Australia. Originally, I planned to include the Arajuno Jungle Lodge in Ecuador, Seed Savers in Decorah, Iowa and the Henry Doorly Zoo and its giant indoor rainforest. While I loved my visit to Seed Savers, it seemed to require a little more massaging into the piece, as it didn't seem logically to go with the other two. While I'm up for that if you really want, I think I'd like to substitute another rainforest for Seed Savers.

I sort of stumbled upon a third rainforest experience while in Australia and it really clicked with my other two experiences. I think I'd like to call the piece, "To the Rainforest Room: A Search for Authenticity in Three Rainforests." The first rainforest was a more or less unmediated experience – if a tree hit me (and it almost did), I'd be dead, plain and simple. The second rainforest was the rainforest at Henry Doorly Zoo, completely mediated and fabricated. I even took a behind-the-scenes look at the rainforest and looked at the plumbing. The third rainforest was sort of in between the other two as far as mediated experience goes. It was in Katoomba, New South Wales, and to get to it, you take the world's steepest funicular railway while the theme song of Indiana Jones blares from a speaker, and then your movements are restricted to a network of boardwalk paths that amble for kilometers. Screens prevent you from leaving the boardwalk to protect the rainforest from you. I was intrigued by a sign at this rainforest which pointed to "The Rainforest Room." And that's where the piece will end. You said it was okay if I'm funny, and yes, I think this will be funny – maybe not belly laughs, but still funny and ironic. I hope you don't mind the slight change from the original, but in the way of these things, my thoughts have really started to gel. I'm pretty excited about it and hope to start the writing now in a few days after I clear my plate just a bit.

All the best, Robin

24 December 2009

Hi Robin,

I trust your command of the material and am on board with the change of plans with this, and thanks for keeping me posted! Take as long as you need. I'll be looking forward to seeing it when you're ready to share.

All the best, holiday cheer, etc., Jennifer

2 February 2010

Hi again, Jennifer,

So, as I mentioned, I'm in France and away from the contract. But if I'm correct, we settled on 4000 words. I'm wondering if there's any wiggle room on that – if I can go up to 5000 or so? The reason I'm asking is that I'm finding that writing about all three rainforests is a little difficult to contain at 4000 words. There's the artificial rainforest I start with in Omaha (the world's largest indoor rainforest), then the rainforest in Ecuador, and finally a rainforest in Australia. The middle rainforest takes up the bulk of the piece. I need about 500 words or so on the final rainforest and my word count going into that is 4500. I'm sure I can cut back some but I'm left with the dilemma of either cutting out the third rainforest (thus rendering the title useless, and I kind of like the title) or cutting back on the second rainforest. If 4000 is what you want, then definitely I'll deliver 4000, but I just wanted to check with you first. Thanks!

All the best, Robin

3 February 2010

Hi Robin,

Word counts at Orion are very fungible. Tell the story the way you want, and we'll work it all out. [Editors' note: the final draft was 5600 words]

Have a croissant pour moi!

Jennifer

8 February 2010
Me again, Jennifer. Sorry to disturb again, but I had meant to add that the direction of the article changed a bit from my original concept to what it has become. While I think/hope it does more or less what I set out to do (in a scenic rather than expositional manner), I'm happy to reconfigure/revise if necessary. I was hoping to keep it subtle and humorous (as we discussed) and avoid making too many Pronouncements about Authenticity. But if we need to add anything, I'm fine with doing so. Of course, I want the piece to be as strong as it can be but I don't have a lot of distance from it yet. All of that is simply to say that I'm flexible . . .

All the best, Robin
[Editors' note: Hemley delivered a draft between this and the following correspondence]

14 May 2010
Dear Jennifer,

I've revised "To the Rainforest Room" because I think it needed context, as in, what is/was at stake for me and how did I come to this subject. The interior of the essay is more or less the same, but I've bookended the essay in a way that I think really adds something important. I hope you'll agree. In any case, please let me know what you think. I'm much happier with this version.

All the best, Robin
15 May 2010

Dear Jennifer,

Okay, very sorry, but you see, I'm in France and last night I dreamed that the French philosopher Jean Baudrillard came to me and complained that he wasn't in my essay. "How can you write about authenticity and not even mention me?" he whined. But he had a point, so I had to at least mention him.

All the best, Robin

17 June 2010
Hi Robin,

Just a quick note to say that I read the latest draft and, hey, this piece keeps getting better without any input from me! Of course, I hope to chime in soon with concrete editorial thoughts, but I figured I'd at least send some kind of smoke signal to tell you what you already know. And thanks for advancing it despite my inability to deal. . .

Jennifer

14 January 2011
Hi Robin,

At long last, I'm sending real, authentic editorial input! I've been to the Rainforest Room and back a bunch of times in the last few days, and I've determined that the story is pretty darn solid. I'm jumping in mostly at the line level, with the occasional margin note of larger significance. I have attached, in PDF form, a real, authentic digital reproduction of the edited manuscript itself.

Overall, the piece walks a really nice line between being playful and delivering salient thoughts. There are a few places where, to my eye, the playfulness either goes over the top or falls flat, and I've marked these as suggested deletions. And it's my feeling that some of the more salient stretches could benefit from some sharpening. I've noted these spots as well.

The third rainforest is the least developed in terms of philosophical takeaways, and perhaps that's appropriate, it having been the one you got for free after buying the other two. But I see room for a little expansion, if you want to set your mind to it.

In the Arajuno Jungle Lodge section, I feel as if some background on the lodge is missing. We never quite get a good picture of what it is, who stays/works there, what kind of mission it has in terms of conservation. There seemed to be a bit too much background on Tom, though, and I found myself unsure as to whether the solar panels warranted as much space as they were given.

Then, in what is perhaps the boldest of my suggestions, I have designated a spot on page 15 as the potential end of the Arajuno section, which would leave a page and a half on the cutting table, including the lemon ants. It's not that I don't like this material. I just feel that it diffuses the point, and that none of it is essential.

See what you think.

In the third rainforest, the landscape description is failing me a little. I can't envision the "ant farm," nor can I really picture how this "attraction" abuts suburbia, though I believe you that it does. You describe very little of the flora and fauna in this rainforest (the Blueberry Ash perhaps being the exception), and I thought saying a little bit more about the nature of the place would help put it in bolder relief, especially against the suburban backdrop. I have suggested an earlier end point to this section as well, but I'm actually not sure either potential ending is really doing what it needs to. You have done too good a job combining wit and unadulterated reality to end on pure comedy. (And the contrived attempt to bring Nebraska back in failed me, though not necessarily because it was contrived.) Which is a long way of saying, can you think a bit more about the ending?

Then, finally, my most important comment on the piece regards the quiz at the end, which I love, in principle, but which has to get way funnier in order to succeed.

This is all by way of suggestion, of course, and for those suggestions you don't fancy, you can certainly stet, or try to imagine something altogether different. I'm just damn glad I accepted this pitch, and grateful that you've been so patient with me. Feel free to call me if you have any questions or want to talk anything over.

If there's any way in hell you can get to this in the next couple weeks, I'd be eternally grateful. (I know, months go by, I don't call, I don't write, and then I want a two-week turnaround!) No one said I didn't have chutzpah . . .

Will you be in DC for AWP?

Cheers, Jennifer

25 January 2011
Hi Jennifer,

I'm officially excited about the essay again. This was the way to go, to re-enter it word by word in my computer. [Editors' note: earlier, Hemley lost his revision in a computer crash.] I was completely able to re-enter the thought processes of the essay as well. I took virtually all of your edits, which I thought were excellent, and I tried to really hone the concepts and make various improvements and adjustments along the way. Please let me know if you think I've succeeded. I added a few paragraphs here and there – I hope they succeed.

Just a caveat: I've tweaked the piece so much that I've lost perspective, so I'm not entirely sure everything I've added works. But I think if not, it's nearly there.

Attached is a photo I hope you can use. If not, I'll get something else.

All the best, Robin

27 January 2011
Hi again, Jennifer,

Sorry to crowd your inbox, but I just had a small fix to a paragraph I wanted to replace in the version you have:

"By "they," he means his neighbor and much bigger reserve, Jatun Sacha. By "chopping block," he means getting shot or blown up. He's found dynamite on the hood of his car before. Last year, a park guard was shot. A bullet grazed his head and when the police came to arrest the man, they found themselves in a standoff with the man's many armed supporters, most of them from Santa Barbara. The police turned and ran."

It's on page 14. I've changed it in my version. This was in response to a query of yours and some fact-checking on my part with Arajuno. Thanks!

Robin

27 January 2011
Dear Jennifer,

I was at a friend's house tonight, chatting about the essay, when all of a sudden, the ending hit me. I think this is it, whether we use the Authenticity quiz or not. Let me know what you think. Can't believe I forgot this until now.

"Half an hour later the Sceniscender, a cable car that fits fifty or so people, lifts me back into the familiar world, past the Three Sisters and a defunct roller coaster that was built over the gorge but has never been put into operation, where I'm delivered into the maw of the inevitable gift shop. Here, I can purchase any number of didgeridoos, placemats, and coffee mugs decorated with aboriginal art, stuffed toy wallabies, and outback hats, all designed, I suppose, to make me feel in touch with something authentic. Resisting it all, I walk outside again, pausing for a moment at a set of statues of three frolicking aboriginals, a man and two women, playing some kind of game that looks like Frisbee, expressions of glee unmistakable on their bronze faces."

Robin

30 January 2011
Dear Robin,

Thanks for the new writing you've done here. I think we're close with this. Another smattering of comments is on the attached.

I hate to say it but I think the bronze statue ending dulls the point you make here, and it feels like it's trying too hard, and asking the reader to do the same. I actually think the piece should end in the inevitable gift shop. So I've proposed a new ending that brings down the dodo graph and a few key sentences from earlier in the piece. See what you think. If you like the general idea, feel free to tinker with the specifics. Oh, and I'm happy to skip the quiz. Save that concept, though. Maybe we can use it again!

If you have time to turn this around before AWP, great. It not, soon thereafter, or the production people will start coming after me.

Cheers, Jennifer

31 January 2011
Hi Jennifer,

This blizzard is worrisome. I've changed my flight twice – I'm going to try rerouting through Dallas, but I have no idea what it's going to be like in Iowa City Wednesday morning. I hope you have smooth travels.

On another note, I don't think I've ever had so much trouble with an ending! But as you say, I think we're close. I tweaked it yet again, slightly. Let me know what you think.

"Here's the test: if you want to replicate it but can't, it's probably authentic. Maybe everything authentic eventually winds up in a museum. Worse, maybe everything authentic eventually winds up depicted on a shot glass in a gift shop. Maybe the very idea of authenticity implies extinction. Authenticity is something to be wished for, catalogued, but never owned. Something to keep at bay our collective nightmares. And that's why I'm in favor of Authenticity."

I just took out a couple of lines that I think were extraneous.

All the best, Robin

1 February 2011
Good luck! I myself am having to bow out of AWP for different reasons.

Whether you get out of Iowa or not, please have a drink in my honor, and I will do the same. I'll be looking over the near final Rainforest Room as time allows. On one of my many drives, I too was thinking that extinction was a real downer of an ending. Happy to see that you've turned that around.

Let's have a phone chat soon!

Jennifer

1 February 2011
Hi Jennifer,

I'm sorry you won't be at AWP, but yes, let's chat soon. I've been thinking more about the Authenticity quiz, making it longer and something that's cumulative, say, "If you live within five miles of an Amish farm, give yourself 2 authenticity points." "If you do Sampoorna Yoga, give yourself three points." "If you do 'Hot Yoga,' take away three points." And so on. I think that would be fun, getting people to think about why they feel good or bad depending on their supposed level of "authenticity."

I'm thinking of using "To the Rainforest Room" as my writing sample for my NEA application this year, actually. I've attached it with the new ending, etc., again just so it's all together. I want to do a whole series of pieces on Authenticity with a book in mind.

Talk soon. All the best, Robin

2 February 2011
Dear Robin,

Here in Mass, our "snowpocalypse" has turned into an unwelcome ice storm. It's grim. Meanwhile, finding the right ending for The Rainforest Room is proving a bit tricky. But first, a few small things along the way:

Tom appears to spell his last name Larson, not Larsen, from the AJL website. Shall we change it? Also, cachama appears to begin with a "c" rather than a "k." And I cannot find any verification that a fish called handia a.) exists, and b.) is indigenous to the Amazon. Can you get me a source?

I changed "In places like this, roads tend to lead to deforestation" to "In jungles like this, roads tend to lead to deforestation."

I changed "My imagination takes flight with this one and I imagine feasts of broiled Kachama with a chonta ragout" to "My imagination takes flight and I envision pan-seared cachama with a chonta ragout."

As for that ending, I think we're getting close. Repeating the first line at the end kind of reminds me of a high school essay, and I think with all the complicated ideas of authenticity that the essay uncovers, it's kind of problematic to end on a simplistic, nearly gleeful "in favor of" sentiment. But I do like the idea of looping back, and want to see what you think of my suggestion below to insert "I am NOT in favor of extinction" after you say "Maybe authenticity implies extinction."

I'm struggling a little with the jogging alongside my nightmares bit but I don't dislike it. I just can't quite figure out how the nightmares relate to the rest of the essay. The nightmare of a world without authenticity? Of a globe full of cheap replicas of trees, landscapes, everything?

As regards the quiz, I am beyond trying to do anything ambitious at the end of the essay (though doing so as a "web extra" might be a possibility). But I can see some value in using just a single multiple-choice question at the end. I dropped one in there from your original, doctored slightly. I'm on the fence. On the one hand, it helps the ending be as light-hearted as the essay, and underscores its main point rather nicely. On the other hand, it could still fall flat, or just be too much. One too many endings? If we can get the jogging alongside nightmares bit to work right, we probably don't need it. But if we leave the jogging out, maybe we can use it instead.

So, for the moment, this is the best I have to offer. See what you think! I'm in. [CAPS]:

> ...And though dodos no longer walk the Earth, I saw a real dodo foot at the British Museum when I was eleven. [I ACTUALLY THINK WE CAN CUT THIS NOW: All those years ago and I never forgot it.]
>
> Maybe everything authentic eventually winds up in [a museum; AN EXHIBIT]. Worse, maybe everything authentic eventually winds up depicted on a shot glass in a gift shop. Maybe the very idea of authenticity implies extinction.
>
> [ADD: For the record, let me state that I am NOT in favor of extinction.]
>
> Here's [the; ONE] test: if you want to replicate it but can't, it's probably authentic. [SO MAYBE] Authenticity is something to be wished for, catalogued, but never owned. Something to keep at bay our collective nightmares [OF WHAT? A WORLD OF CHEAP REPLICAS DEVOID OF ANYTHING GENUINE?]. [But that's not so bad; RIGHT NOW I'M THINKING THAT A MESSY DEFINITION OF AUTHENTICITY IS BETTER THAN A WORLD UTTERLY DEVOID OF ANYTHING AUTHENTIC.] I'd rather be inside the exhibit than
>
> jogging alongside my nightmares.
>
> [CUT: And that's why I'm in favor of Authenticity.]
>
> [I'M ON THE FENCE ABOUT ADDING THIS:]
>
> And now, for review purposes, I'd like to close with a multiple-choice question.

If a road is built in the rainforest, it will inevitably lead to (mark all that apply):

a. Deforestation
b. Ushito's re-election
c. A store that sells Easy Cheese
d. Nebraska

Don't send me another Word doc at this point. I've already reformatted the piece to go to copyedit. If we can stick to email from here that would be great.

Thanks!
All the best, Jennifer

2 February 2011
Dear Jennifer,

Thanks! You're right about Tom's name. Stupid mistake. Not sure how I did that. I'm checking with him right now about the fish. I suspect they're native names. I'm mulling over the other suggestions, but I'm mostly on board, I think. Stay tuned. Just spent the morning shoveling snow!

All the best, Robin

2 February 2011
Hi Jennifer,

I like the one question quiz, but if we're going to restore it, then let's also restore this line in the intro: "And so I present for your further confusion if not edification, three rainforests. At the end of this essay, you will be given a short quiz."

Thanks, Robin

2 February 2011
Sure. Just so I'm clear, are you still mulling over the ending in general?

Jennifer

3 February 2011
Hi Jennifer,

Okay, I THINK I've got it. I've taken most of your suggestions and tried to clarify the end. I THINK the last paragraph nails it. I hope so. Ending with an image from the essay is best, I think.

I like the quiz, but I can go either way. Do you think it might undercut the power of the end now that (hopefully) the ending is more powerful, but not hopeless?

Here it is. I'll be eager for your thoughts.

Stepping back outside into the parking lot, I find myself thinking about how often our idea of what's real differs from what's actually there. And about how certain concepts persist in our consciousness long after they've disappeared. When the Dutch killed the last Dodo on Mauritius in the 1600s, the idea of the Dodo did not cease to exist. It became the poster bird for all creatures who are too stupid to save themselves. Still, any loss over time becomes more bearable. I can't authentically experience a Dodo, but I can imagine one. I can Google a dodo and, in this sense, get closer to a Dodo than most people did who were alive when dodos still existed. And though dodos no longer walk the Earth, I saw a real Dodo foot at the British Museum when I was eleven.

Maybe everything authentic eventually winds up an exhibit. Worse, maybe everything authentic eventually winds up depicted on a shot glass in a gift shop. Maybe the very idea of authenticity implies impending extinction. For the record: I'm not in favor of extinction. Here's one test: if you want to replicate it but can't, it's probably authentic.

So maybe authenticity is something to be wished for, catalogued, but never owned. Something we can't quite pin down, but nevertheless yearn for.

Something to keep at bay a while longer our collective nightmare of a globe full of polyurethane trees and wild animals clocking out for the evening.

And now, for review purposes, I'd like to close with a multiple-choice question.

If a road is built in the rainforest, it will inevitably lead to (mark all that apply):

a.   Deforestation
b.   Ushito's re-election
c.   A store that sells Easy Cheese
d.   Nebraska

Robin Hemley

3 February 2011
Hi Robin,

I'm mostly with you here. Would you consider changing this:

Something to keep at bay a while longer our collective nightmare of a globe full of polyurethane trees and wild animals clocking out for the evening.

to this?:

Something that, for a while anyway, can keep at bay the nightmare of a globe covered with polyurethane trees and inhabited by wild animals who clock out every evening.

I do think we leave the quiz on the cutting table. Unless you want to try to do something online.

Are we there yet?
And by the way, did you make it to DC?

Thanks for bearing with me on this until the not-so-bitter end. . .

Jennifer

3 February 2011
Hi Jennifer,

Virtual high-five! I think we're there. I'm with you on the proposed change! Phew. Haven't made it yet to DC! Still trying. My next attempt is tonight. Yes, let's leave the quiz on the cutting-room floor. Thanks for bearing with ME. I'm usually really pretty good with endings, but this was a tough one.

Robin

12 February 2011
Dear Robin,

I got Rainforest Room back from the copyeditor, and there's nothing of substance worth reporting back to you. Mostly house style stuff. The one thing I wanted to raise with you, though, is capitalization. Before sending the piece to copyedit, I studied the use of capitalization with regard to "Authentic" and "Authenticity," and tried to make it as consistent, and effective, as possible. I really like the tongue-in-cheek use of capitalization, but as I worked towards applying it in any systematic sort of way, it was hard to know just where to draw the line: Do we capitalize all uses of "authentic" and "authenticity" in the first section of the piece? What about the final section? What about "authentically" or "inauthentic"? And then there were the occasional capitalized phrases placed in juxtaposition with "Authentic" and "Authenticity," such as the "Real Thing," and "Place and People." I really like these too.

The copyeditor understood right away the dilemma over when to apply capitalization, and gave two suggestions for how to apply it consistently. As I studied her suggestions, I realized that I didn't like their implications. Any systematic application of capitalization risks overusing it, or putting emphasis in places where you don't actually want it.

So here's where I think we are left: apply capitalization somewhat idiosyncratically, or don't use it at all. I was surprised to find, when I looked at the piece without any capitalization of these phrases, that I didn't miss it all that much. The narrative intentions are not lost at all, though it does make the piece a tad less playful. I'm attaching the final Word doc as I have it now, sans capitals, to see what you think. I wouldn't mind restoring some of the capitalization to preserve the playfulness, though it would thrust us right back into that dilemma of how widely to apply it.

I'm sure this must seem ridiculously nit-picky. And with everything I've got going on right now it seems sort of silly, in a way. But we editors pride ourselves on being able to justify every aspect of the stories we publish, and this is proving a little slippery.

I'm eager to hear what you think!

Jennifer

12 February 2011
Hi Jennifer,

Wow, how nit-picky! No, just kidding. I'm grateful for the close attention. I find it impressive, actually. So, I think I have a very simple fix. Everything you pointed out makes a lot of sense. My feeling is that we can have it both ways if we simply capitalize in the beginning and at the very end, capitalizing the word "Extinction" too. Here's the beginning:

> I'm in favor of Authenticity. Maybe I should rephrase that. I want everything in my life to be Authentic. I want to only eat Authentic Food and only have Authentic Experiences. When I travel, I want to travel Authentically (hot air balloon, camel, steam railway). I want to meet Authentic People (family

farmers, I think, are authentic; people you meet in the Polka Barn at the Iowa State Fair; members of lost tribes; chain-smoking hair dressers named Betty). I want to think Authentic Thoughts.

And here's the end:

Maybe everything Authentic eventually winds up an exhibit. Worse, maybe everything Authentic eventually winds up depicted on a shot glass in a gift shop. Maybe the very idea of Authenticity implies Extinction. For the record, I'm not in favor of Extinction. Here's one test: if you want to replicate it but can't, it's probably Authentic. So maybe Authenticity is something to be wished for, catalogued, but never owned. Something we can't quite pin down, but nevertheless yearn for. Something that, for a while anyway, can keep at bay the nightmare of a globe covered with polyurethane trees and inhabited by wild animals who clock out every evening.

Everything else would remain lower case except perhaps the subtitle. What do you think? That retains some of the whimsy, but doesn't force it to be annoyingly consistent.

All the best, Robin

14 February 2011
Hi Robin,

Thanks for proposing something simple! I've mulled it over, and I agree that restoring the caps in the first graph is a good way to preserve the fun without overdoing it. I'm less sure about the final graph. The tone there is more serious, and I think the playful caps there sort of undercut the takeaway.

Having the benefit of your suggestion, my instinct is to actually do more with these semi-rhetorical caps in the first section, and then not doing any more after that. Along those lines, here's what I'd propose:

I'm in favor of Authenticity.
Maybe I should rephrase that.

I want everything in my life to be Authentic. I want to only eat Authentic Food and only have Authentic Experiences. When I travel, I want to travel authentically (hot air balloon, camel, steam railway). I want to meet Authentic People (family farmers, I think, are authentic; people you meet in the Polka Barn at the Iowa State Fair; members of lost tribes; chain-smoking hair dressers named Betty). I want to think Authentic Thoughts.

Actually, Authenticity baffles me...

...

The Tasaday were neither Authentic Cavemen nor a hoax. . .

. . .

Nature declawed, stuffed, mounted. What then do we really want from the Authentic Destinations of our imaginations? And how do our perceptions of them differ from the Real Thing? When we think of an unspoiled. . .

. . .

My experience with the Tasaday has rendered me hyperaware of the aura of desperation and melancholy surrounding our common need for the Authentic, especially in regard to Place and People. Call it a sixth sense. . ..

And that's it. What do you think? I sure am glad you're flattered by nit-pickery. . .

Jennifer

26 April 2012
Dear Robin,

We were just informed that "To the Rainforest Room" won a Pushcart, and will appear in the next Pushcart anthology, which has some long Roman numeral to distinguish it from its predecessors. I'm super psyched. I was hoping it would get noticed.
  Rah rah!

Jennifer

26 April 2012
Oh my God! How absolutely fantastic!! And I'm hard at work on my new one. You made my day!! Yay!

Robin

Conversation with Robin Hemley and jennifer Sahn

The editors

First of all, thank you for sharing the entire archive of documents, which shows in great detail the entire process of the writing of this amazing essay. This piece has a slightly different genesis from others we have examined. Jennifer, you first accepted Robin's pitch, and over a two-month period, this initial pitch was put through a kind of intramural edit as the reach of the project responded to new possibilities and connections. We can see from your first answer to Robin that even though the story has not yet been commissioned, you offer some guidelines as to what kind of story would fit the magazine:

  This kind of piece can be pretty hard to pitch, and equally hard to commission, because success lies almost entirely in the execution. But if we are talking about a literary sort of narrative, grounded in scene and setting, with a solid "think piece" center, then I am pretty interested.

Could you briefly tell us what attracted you to the first pitch? How much direction do you tend to give at this more conceptual stage, where the writer-editor relationship exists in a state of potentiality, almost entirely based on a faith in the promise of the blank page rather than something more tangible?

And Robin, it is clear that you needed to make a decision before the writing has even started. It may very well be that this was the type of text you intended to write, which makes the decision easier, but still, what we see is that some form of editing process is already taking shape.

Sahn

I'm attracted to stories that are surprising from the outset, that take up an original subject or take an original approach to a familiar subject, stories that are searching for answers but don't promise to necessarily find them. Robin's story seemed to be firmly planted in the center of this Venn diagram, so my first instinct was, *Hell, yes!* But before that, I needed to make sure the author and I were on the same page about what kind of journey we were embarking upon – which we were, or at least seemed to be.

When a pitch or a draft catches my eye, I will give the author as little or as much input as I think necessary in order to communicate how I think the piece could be improved, and/or how it might need to evolve to fit the publication to which it's been offered. Sometimes this involves a conversation about framing or scope, but certainly not always. This piece, a narrative essay that's partly reported but largely conceptual, is not the kind of story that's easy for an author to pitch, or for an editor to accept on the basis of a pitch, and it evolved a lot during the months that we were working on it. The editorial process works best when both parties are passionate, open-minded, and unafraid of where the journey will take them.

As you can see from the correspondence, this was my first time working with Robin Hemley. He was essentially an unknown author to me at the time. I saw in his pitch a strong voice, combined with intellectual curiosity and an ability to write sentences that are a pleasure to read. When you choose to work with a writer for the first time, there's risk involved, but this story was well worth it, and Robin had already won two Pushcart Prizes, so he was obviously someone who is capable of great things.

Hemley

I've worked with a number of editors before and I like the editorial process a lot. I believe I'm an enthusiastic collaborator in the process when I have a good editor behind me, and I'm always open to good ideas, even when they don't originate with me. I certainly see it as helpful when an editor gives me an idea of what they're looking for, especially when I'm writing for a magazine with a particular kind of vision. If you've already made the decision to write for a magazine with its particular style, you need to have an idea of what they're looking for. So, when Jennifer said, "Scene," and "think piece," I thought, "Okay, I've got this."

The editors

Robin, the numerous drafts you sent us show your thinking processes before the editor began working on the text as such, but this does not entail a lack of editorial input. Your email correspondence with Jennifer offers a great deal of fascinating insights, from the changes in direction and adding new ideas, concerns about the length, the struggle to find the right ending, nitpicking, etc. Often, it looks like you only needed some support from the editor to try out an idea that struck you while you were doing research or just travelling. What particularly stands out is the message where you think you are about to change direction in the way you envision the story, and this is related to Jennifer's early comment on what kind of story she would be fine with:

> You said it was okay if I'm funny, and yes, I think this will be funny – maybe not belly laughs, but still funny and ironic. I hope you don't mind the slight change from the original, but in the way of these things, my thoughts have really started to gel. I'm pretty excited about it and hope to start the writing now in a few days after I clear my plate just a bit.
>
> . . .
>
> I had meant to add that the direction of the article changed a bit from my original concept to what it has become. While I think/hope it does more or less what I set out to do (in a scenic rather than expositional manner), I'm happy to reconfigure/revise if necessary. I was hoping to keep it subtle and humorous (as we discussed), and avoid making too many Pronouncements about Authenticity. But if we need to add anything, I'm fine with doing so. Of course, I want the piece to be as strong as it can be but I don't have a lot of distance from it yet. All of that is simply to say that I'm flexible . . .

Can you say something about this part of the process?

Hemley

I'm always a bit vulnerable in my writing, and yes, sometimes what I need is permission, whether it's from myself or an editor. As I mentioned, the piece had indeed shifted and there were elements that I had originally wanted to report on that just hadn't panned out. For instance, I had wanted to visit Seed Savers, a famous "seed vault" in Dekorah, Iowa, which for many years had been collecting heirloom varieties of seeds. I did

indeed drive up to Dekorah and interview one of the founders and the current director and I found myself in the middle of another story, equally interesting, but different.
The founding couple of Seed Savers had divorced and had a rather nasty falling out
about the direction of Seed Savers, with one side accusing the other of being in the
pocket of Monsanto. And when I brought it up, the director became defensive and a
little angry and I thought, "This is a great story for 60 Minutes, but not for me." I had
wanted mostly to talk to them about the notion of "authentic" seeds, but I saw that the
other story, the one they didn't want to tell me, was too tempting. If I spent any more
time around them, I'd think I was an investigative reporter and really get derailed. So,
I cut Seed Savers out and starting focusing on the piece I was writing about the notion
of rain forest – something I knew a little more about, in any case.

The editors

"To the Rainforest Room" is a creative non-fiction story that takes *authenticity*
(defining it, locating it) as its central theme. Given that the most precarious element
of the editing process is arguably the maintenance of a balance between preserving
the raw, authorial voice – the *primary aesthetic* – and the more detached fine-tuning
necessary for publication, we might see this "search" as being a broader metaphor
for editing as a practice. This brings about certain areas we are interested in exploring:
commitment to theme, changes of direction, voice. But first, can you say something
about your approach to this *primary aesthetic*?

Sahn

Part of an editor's job is to preserve the author's voice. This is a fundamental facet of
the writer-editor relationship. There are no parts of the editorial process to which
this rule does not apply. Also, this is how you earn a writer's trust. Over time, the
more you work with an author, the more intimate you become with their style, the
easier this gets. The editor is the invisible partner. Any words that he or she has added
(and sometimes this is a lot), should be un-discernable (even to the writer, upon
looking back on the piece weeks or months later). The best editorial journeys are a
sort of collective groping in the dark for the best way to say something, the best way
to generate a reader experience that is all-consuming, lacking in a single glitch, speed
bump, or turn of phrase that could cause a reader to fall out of the spell of the story.

Hemley

It's a fair point and sometimes I think editors can get a little carried away with
changes. There are several instances I can think of, at least once in a magazine piece
and once in a book, when I felt my own voice was lost because of an editorial
change I acquiesced to and shouldn't have. That's my own fault of course, but when
and if I ever run across the offensive passages, or simply recall them, I wince, thinking,
I would never say it that way.

The editors

"To the Rainforest Room" was revised and restructured three times before the first concrete editorial overhaul. Notably, this first key draft includes an introductory meditation on the merits of Cheese Whiz and a pop quiz by way of conclusion, both of which are either cut, changed, or compressed in the final edit. Robin, in the correspondence, you talk about these sections as *bookends* that create context and add something important, something that illuminates what was at stake and how you came to the process, or, implicitly, what fundamentally motivates the piece. Certainly, some of the most substantial of editorial changes occur in these bookends. Robin, thinking first of Part One, could you talk about how these sections initially shaped the direction of the piece, and the impact of the revisions (proposed and effected) on that context. Did the "something important" itself change as the edits revealed new layers of narrative connection and cohesion?

Hemley

I can't remember how the pop quiz started, but I think Jennifer suggested it or the two of us came up with the idea during a phone conversation. I'm often whimsical and a little silly and so I liked this idea. We later thought maybe we'd put the quiz on *Orion*'s website, but that eventually passed, too. I think I just needed to get the truly silly ideas out of my head, though Cheez Whiz, which remains, is pretty silly in itself. I think I wanted to mock the idea of authenticity a little, not merely the idea of Cheez Whiz itself, which is hardly worth mocking, but even the idea of authentic cheddar cheese made in caves in Cheddar, England, within 48 kilometers of Wells Cathedral. I'm really mocking myself and those like me who have no idea why Wells Cathedral is important to the making of cheddar cheese, but who like the sound of this anyway. The problem is that I'm a sucker for lines like this because I know that only four counties in Southwest England are allowed to designate their cheese as "West County Farmhouse cheddar cheese." That's almost unbearably authentic, it's irresistible, and I'm a bit of a fool for thinking so. I can't help but think that there's some training involved in this search for authenticity that we should resist, especially when it comes down to marketing and what we think will make us more special and what won't, especially when it comes to taste. We just have to remember that lobster until the late 19th century was considered in the U.S. at least a food fit for prisoners and not the delicacy many people think of it as today. The lobster didn't change. We did.

The editors

An editorial focus that applies to the piece as a whole concerns *voice*: the level of colloquialism, the accuracy of cultural references, the length and tone of various asides. Let us look at a few examples:

The second sentence, key in that it supports the central quest for Authenticity, vacillates from "Let me rephrase that" to "Um, let me rephrase that" to "Maybe I should rephrase that." Then, Baudrillard, whom you added to the text after a bizarre dream you had (mentioned in one of the emails) is deemed an "overly intellectual escape-hatch from Cheese Whiz-dom," and cut. Then we see how Cheese Whiz – following Sahn's comment "Cheez Whiz comes in a jar. Easy Cheese comes in that can with the nozzle – and don't ask how I know this!" – becomes Easy Cheese, and is even promoted to the subject of Part One's title. "Florets" of Cheese Whiz become "swathes" or "blobs," and finally "florets" again.

In some ways, all these changes could appear insignificant, yet in others they are key to the overall impact of the piece, and more than once your correspondence or margin notes identify the need for authenticity here too, particularly in maintaining what you describe as its integral *whimsy* and *playfulness*. Jennifer, you observe, in one of the messages, that the first key draft of the piece "walks a really nice line between being playful and delivering salient thoughts" but also that there are "a few places where … the playfulness either goes over the top or falls flat," and you mark those for deletion.

Sahn

One way to make a story better is to cut any nonessential parts that are simply not working, whether it's because they undermine or dilute the main idea, are too much of a distraction, or otherwise gum up the works. Sometimes it's the editor's job to save a writer from him or herself. Most good writers recognize this. They want to be saved. It's like when a friend tells you your tag is showing, or your partner says you have something in your teeth. Writers rely on editors to show them what they can't see.

An editor wants to publish the strongest, shortest, most potent and moving version of a story. Sometimes the writer and editor have the luxury of months or years in which to get there. Other times, not. This story wasn't commissioned for a specific issue of the magazine. In fact, I never even showed it to anybody else at the magazine until I knew it was one or two drafts away from being the best I thought it could be. Robin and I had the luxury of time to obsess over details, largely to good effect. I find that last stretch of the editorial process, the finest of fine-tuning, to be uniquely satisfying.

Hemley

I rely heavily on my editor's ear for what sounds right and what falls flat or goes over the top. I tend to take a lot of risks, and sometimes those risks are shots in the dark. Will this work? Won't it? There's only one way to find out, and that's what the editor's there for, in part. Humor, especially, is tricky, and I'm aware that I can sometimes be excessive, but sometimes the bits that I worry might be excessive turn out to be worth the risk. But yes, an awful lot of work goes into deciding whether "florets" works better than "swathes" or "blobs." For some reason, it does work better, perhaps because it's such an elegant sounding word in opposition to Easy

Cheese. You'd think we were creating little museum pieces the way we slave over a word choice. In the scheme of things, no one would have noticed or cared if we had settled on the word "blobs," but maybe if the editor isn't a perfectionist then she'll start to get lazy and will let other things more important slip by her.

The editors

Specifically, the ending is clearly more problematic, particularly in regard to the Authenticity quiz, which does not feature in the published version, although there is a real sense of fondness for it throughout both the correspondence and the draft trail. The alternative ending returns to the Sceniscender of Katoomba and concludes on these lines:

> Resisting it all, I walk outside again, pausing for a moment at a set of statues of three frolicking aboriginals, a man and two women, playing some kind of game that looks like Frisbee, expressions of glee unmistakable on their bronze faces.

This ending presents its own difficulties. Jennifer, you express the concern here that it is "trying too hard, and asking the reader to do the same." In an email you write: "I'm actually not sure either potential ending is really doing what it needs to. You have done too good a job combining wit and unadulterated reality to end on pure comedy." Do you feel it was the commitment to authenticity as a theme that made the conclusion so difficult to get right? What is it exactly that you felt that ending needed to do? Would you have insisted on the cut if Robin had not made it himself?

And Robin, did you know all along that the ending was not quite right and that you would, eventually, have to change it? Jennifer shows much patience, so the question is also how would a more brash editor, like Gordon Lish, affect the entire process. You got a chance to try it out and arrive at the same conclusion as Jennifer in a more relaxed way.

Sahn

The ending is crucial to any story because it is the thing that resonates in the reader's mind as he or she turns the page, gets up from the couch, goes off to cook dinner, or out for a walk. A good ending is the verbal equivalent of flash of lightning or a sucker punch to the gut. Or, in this case, a crystallization of the story's inherent dilemma, placing the onus on the reader to make his or her own determination for what it all means. The emotional stakes are high. Do we want to leave the reader feeling hopeful, worried, enlightened, inspired?

With this story, there was an ever-present risk of over-trivializing the idea of authenticity. But I also knew there was no neat and tidy ending where everything would be explained. In my estimation, the story needed an ending that reinforced the rigor and light-heartedness of the inquiry but stopped short of a making any kind of declaration. In some ways, this story scratches the surface of one of life's greatest conundrums: what is real and what is fake; what should we value and what should we consider disposable? I wanted readers to walk away thinking about these complexities and applying that thinking to whatever they are facing in their own lives.

As for the quiz, I remember having a lot of fun with it during our email exchanges. It was almost like a game we were playing while we were working on the story. I don't remember being concerned about whether or not it would end up in the story. I guess at some point we decided that it wouldn't.

To be clear, though, I never insist on anything. Ultimately, it's the writer's name going on the piece. It's my job to make recommendations. If I do a good job articulating why I'm making them, I've done my job. It's up to the writer to decide what to do from there. I've had very few writers dig in their heels over anything. I usually pick up the phone at that point, because I realize that I've missed something essential about what the author is trying to do. If I understand the author's objective, I can help make it happen. Good communication is essential to making good editorial choices.

Hemley

Was I really that strident about keeping it? I don't remember it that way. Lish almost WAS my editor for my first collection of stories. He accepted it and then unaccepted it a week later for reasons only known to him. I'll never know how I would have reacted. I probably would have rolled over.

Endings, anyway, are difficult and it's easy to kill an otherwise wonderful essay or story with the wrong ending. I knew where I wanted to end, just not how. I suppose the quiz must have become a little darling, though it's funny that I don't remember it that way now. I have no idea why I was so attached to it.

The editors

There is one thing which seems to fall into what you both call nitpicking, but which ultimately is anything but: the capitalization of the word "authenticity" and other phrases. Jennifer, you could have told Robin you didn't like it and that it was not necessary, but you elaborate in some detail what should be done:

> One thing I wanted to raise with you, though, is capitalization. Before sending the piece to copyedit, I studied the use of capitalization with regard to "Authentic" and "Authenticity," and tried to make it as consistent, and effective, as possible. I really like the tongue-in-cheek us of capitalization, but as I worked towards applying it in any systematic sort of way, it was hard to know just where to draw the line: Do we capitalize all uses of "authentic" and "authenticity" in the first section of the piece? What about the final section? What about "authentically" or "inauthentic"? And then there were the occasional capitalized phrases placed in juxtaposition with "Authentic" and "Authenticity," such as the "Real Thing," and "Place and People." I really like these too.

The copyeditor understood right away the dilemma over when to apply capitalization, and gave two suggestions for how to apply it consistently. As I studied her suggestions, I realized that I didn't like their implications. Any systematic application of capitalization risks overusing it, or putting emphasis in places where you don't actually want it.

So here's where I think we are left: apply capitalization somewhat idiosyncratically, or don't use it at all. I was surprised to find, when I looked at the piece without any capitalization of these phrases, that I didn't miss it all that much. The narrative intentions are not lost at all, though it does make the piece a tad less playful.

We find the point about idiosyncrasy essential here. It offers Robin space for decision, and brings forth the unique authenticity of his project.

Sahn

There is style and there is grammar and sometimes the two are in conflict. I tend to choose style over grammar because I care more about voice than following rules. Copyeditors are trained grammarians, but editors sometimes choose to overrule them. The copyeditor in this case was doing her job by pointing out the inconsistency. And yet it was clear to me that there was no consistent way to deal with the capitalization here that would generate the best reader experience. We were very far off the map in terms of the *Chicago Manual of Style*. We were left with our gut feelings. Those are usually the best feelings, the most authentic feelings. You are right, there is something about our diligence with getting this story right that is reflective of its subject. But this story didn't earn that level of scrutiny because of its subject. All stories should be authentic stories. All stories should be told in the best way possible.

Hemley

Isn't it marvelous how Jennifer strikes this wonderfully meditative tone in her comments that's at once wise, self-interrogating, sure-footed, and flattering? You're right in that she leaves a lot of room for me to make a decision, but she's also asking me to think more deeply about the piece, to engage more deeply and fully understand my choices and why I've made them. I think this is what a great editor does. It can seem brutal at times the way a hard massage can be brutal. You're a little bruised but you feel so much better afterwards.

The editors

Jennifer, taking a particular look at Part Three: Arajuno Jungle Lodge, Ecuador, we would like to consider what you say is "perhaps the boldest of [your] suggestions." You write:

> I have designated a spot . . . as the potential end of the Arajuno section, which would leave a page and a half on the cutting table, including the lemon ants.

It's not that I don't like this material. I just feel that it diffuses the point, and that none of it is essential . . .

Why did you make this suggestion? How do you decide what is essential?

Sahn

Part of earning the trust of the reader involves staying on topic, and not veering off into territory that doesn't really advance the story you are trying to tell. This long section went too far afield, in my opinion. If it's not helping the story to succeed, then it is just making the story longer, its message more diffuse. I'm a lover of longform, but I also believe every sentence needs to earn its place. Cutting entire sections or pages full of text is sometimes necessary. But I'm mindful that the initial impact of seeing that big X through a page of text is probably a little painful for an author. By mentioning it in the cover note, and acknowledging that it's a significant suggestion, I'm preparing the writer. *Brace for impact. This might hurt a bit.*

The editors

Robin, in an email, you write:

> I'm in France and last night I dreamed that the French philosopher Jean Baudrillard came to me and complained that he wasn't in my essay."How can you write about authenticity and not even mention me?" he whined. But he had a point, so I had to at least mention him.

Although Baudrillard did not end up making the final cut, there is something in this that perhaps is not always talked about: an implication that editing is an ephemeral, instinctive process as much as it as an externalized, concrete, and objective one.

Hemley

Yes, editing is probably much like the writing process, essaying the essay, as it were. I think the key concept here is "experience." An experienced editor will be judging the manuscript at hand based on her experience with hundreds of other edited manuscripts over her career. She also knows her audience and knows what will work for them and what won't, and so in this sense the editing is objective. It might seem intuitive, but it's a long, learned process.

The editors

We would like to consider wider issues of editing that seem exposed by the central themes of the essay, which poses this question of the environment: "How much do we need to strip away before we reach the desired level of Authenticity?" It seems applicable to the editing process too. You could go as far as to say the observation of the truly authentic "moment of disregard" that closes Part Two acts as a reminder that a final draft is in some ways as artificial and carefully constructed as the Lied Rainforest of Nebraska. The finished piece is its own kind of illusion: it needs to feel un-tampered with – which takes us back to Gottlieb's notion of the editor as *the invisible hand* – but almost always requires the literary equivalent of the Lied's wading pools and reverse-osmosis system to find its most authentic rendering. It is, as the story goes, "Planned to look unplanned." Does editing become an act of ventriloquism?

Hemley

Sometimes, yes, editing can be an act of ventriloquism, but only in those instances when the writer has really relinquished full control, moments he or she might later regret. The idea of ventriloquism is a bit troubling to me. A good editor is trying to catch the moments that seem inauthentic, leading the writer to a close reexamination of his work, which should render ventriloquism unnecessary. But I tend to question the word "authentic" when it comes to language or "voice." As you point out, the authentic voice, whatever that is, is created artificially. It, too, is a simulacrum designed to sound "natural." Authenticity is a means, not an end, at least in the realm of the written.

Sahn

To make good suggestions, an editor needs to channel the writer, to walk for a while in his or her shoes, to generate phrases that the writer himself would generate, to know what fits organically and what sticks out like a sore thumb. A talented and trustworthy editor should be able to make suggestions that feel authentic to the writer, that sometimes even impress the writer by being so perfectly suited to what the writer had meant to say and how he or she might have hoped to say it. This is an act of caretaking: of paying attention, reading closely, and thinking deeply about word choice. Done well, it's the ultimate form of flattery.

As far as command of the material – what to keep, what to jettison, how to string the pieces together into a coherent whole – it is, in a very real way, a conscious effort to manipulate the reader. You are trying to generate a certain experience, and you will make a hundred different choices towards that end. Niagara Falls was so extensively engineered (rocks shaped and water channeled) that no part of it can conceivably be considered natural today. That may be a good metaphor for storytelling.

The editors

A broad question regarding authenticity. Personally, we do not think that the kind and level of input you, Jennifer, give Robin creates a sense of inauthenticity. On the contrary, we would argue that authenticity arises from this type of collaboration rather than being some form of singular creation performed in isolation. Human beings share stories and the very act of writing is about sharing, about exposing yourself, about shaping yourself through interaction. It is, as Jean-Luc Nancy (to mention another French philosopher) said about love, that it is to give what you do not have, and what you do not have is your (authentic) self, because the self is created through communication.

In contrast, famously, Gordon Lish's editorial relationship with Raymond Carver often faces accusations of compromising authorial authenticity. The restoration of the stories to Carver's originals in *Beginners* – stripped free of Lish's edits – presents a more authentic experience, and yet not necessarily one we prefer. The Easy Cheese question seems pertinent here too: "How can we hope to live authentically when we have been compromised by prior experience?" How can we hope to read authentically when the editing process, by definition, compromises (or dilutes) that by layering in multiple voices to the final piece?

Sahn

A writer's journals or notepads are the feedstock for essays and stories. The stories themselves necessarily involve manipulation: on the part of the editor, surely, but also – and much more significantly – on the part of the writer. I take issue with the word *compromise* – and *dilute* – as well as the idea that an editor is layering his or her own voice on top of the writer's. People who see editing this way either don't understand the fine art of it, or they have had too many experiences with bad editors. Bad editors exist. Avoid them if you can.

Hemley

Okay, now I get what you mean by ventriloquism. I think I agree that what's most collaborative can seem most authentic, and also what seems most contradictory. As Blake writes, "Do what you will this Life's a fiction/And is made up of contradiction."

Theoretical Trigger Warning: I'm going to talk about Roland Barthes here.

While I don't agree completely with Barthes' famous assertion that every text is so collaborative as to have no essential author, I agree with it, too. His famous quote, "The text is a tissue of quotations drawn from innumerable centers of culture," feels more like one Zeno's paradoxes than what we actually experience in our reading lives. Texts are embodied and subjective, but they are also drawn from innumerable centers of culture. The editor's voice is one more tissue, maybe many tissues, that are added to the text to make it seem authored by a singular person. Is that contradictory? Well, yes, it's meant to be.

The editors

Jennifer, your edit strikes a great balance between what we could see as straightforward cuts, changes, and suggestions. In the first email commentary, you write:

"This is all by way of suggestion, of course, and for those suggestions you don't fancy, you can certainly stet, or try to imagine something altogether different." In the actual edit, sometimes you just cross out pieces of text, add or exchange phrases, and sometimes you put suggestions (marked by the recurring question mark) even though in most places your alternatives do read as the better options. Often the cut is not made, but rather suggested, if you are concerned with a long piece of text, an entire paragraph, as for instance when you write: "this feels to me like a really strong end to the Arajuno section. What follows, mostly seems to draw things out. Unnecessarily. Can you imagine parting with the next page and a half."

Is this related to the potential sensitivity of the author to sheer cutting or do you really mean it is optional whether or not the cut is made? The sense we get is that you would insist on a cut and would be ready to argue for it but hope the simple note like "not essential" will suffice. The section in Part Three about Larsen is an interesting example because there you suggest a longer cut but it is clear from your note that it is not enough, that the paragraph needs condensing, and you are not going to do it for him.

Sahn

Editing, like anything, really, requires diplomacy. That means having opinions, but being open to the possibility that someone else may have a better idea. It means acknowledging that there is a human being on the other end of the correspondence who has already thought deeply about everything on the page. All of my edits are always by way of suggestion. I don't think editing by insistence would be respectful, nor do I think it would lead to a better product. We are giving directions, but we are not driving the car.

Hemley

I saw this as a real dialogue, not as a ginger means of trying to get me to do her bidding, though I suppose if that's indeed what she wanted, it worked. I never had a sense that Jennifer was coy in her suggestions. When she asked, "Can you imagine?" she was being respectful, though there was an implied, "You need to defend this section if you want to keep it." This part of the editing process can be a bit frustrating because you feel like a student who needs to get an "A" but doesn't know what the teacher wants! *Just tell me! I need an A.* But here's the thing: *The editor doesn't know either what you need to get an "A."* All she knows is *Not this.* It's always up to the author to figure it out and this is where I love to rise to the challenge. I once wrote a piece for *New York Magazine* and they told me that the piece I turned in was not what they had expected at all and if I wanted to get it in the magazine, I had to rewrite the entire article in the next 24 hours. But I was at a writers' conference at the time, and I was expected that day to do a three-hour workshop, give a lecture and then a reading. My duties ended at 9 pm with 12 hours to go. After my reading, I loaded up on junk food (the story was about summer camp so junk food seemed appropriate), went back to my hotel room and wrote the damn thing again. What led me into the new and better version was their outright dismay over the first version and an opening that I came up with that set the tone for the rest of the piece and allowed me to crystalize what it was I needed to discover in writing the piece. Fear of failure and frustration sometimes inspire an authentic voice. In any case, I love moments like that, at least in hindsight. Sometimes, you're just in combat with a piece, and you just have to show it who's boss.

The editors

Robin, in one of the messages towards the end of the writing and editing process, after your hard drive crashed and you had to type up the entire piece from a pdf file, you write:

> I've tweaked the piece so much that I've lost perspective, so I'm not entirely sure everything I've added works … This was the way to go, to re-enter it word by word in my computer. I was completely able to re-enter the thought processes of the essay as well.

What you express here is the risk artists run following a desire to perfect their work, the risk of over-editing, or editing a story to pieces. How do you know when to stop? Is it instinctive, or do you have tips for beginners how to develop this instinct?

Hemley

What I see here is my own exhaustion. This is exactly what I'm talking about. Writing is hard enough and then your hard drive crashes. But okay, just view that as a new opportunity to enter the text. But no, you're sick of the text. Wouldn't it be nice to just write back to Jennifer and ask her for a kill fee and use it to buy a nice bottle of scotch? I was an exchange student in Japan when I was seventeen, and the phrase I loved the most was "Gambatte" which means "keep trying" or "don't give up." So, I say "Gambatte" to the essay. Bring it on. When I stop is when the essay and I have exhausted one another, when we face off, bow, and walk away. I have no tips for beginners except to *always think of yourself as a beginner.*

Sahn

A story is never really done. Once in a rare while I feel confident that a story is the best version of itself that I can help it to be. Mostly, though, there is a moment when it is due to fact-check, to copyedit, when galleys are circulating and you're no longer able to make changes. Sometimes, at the last minute possible, you magically figure out how to fix something that wasn't working. I don't think there's such a thing as *over-editing*. I think what you are talking about is *bad editing*. On the other hand, there have been suggestions that I've made that I have questioned after the fact. Sometimes I reverse myself: I un-suggest something I had previously suggested. There is no ego in it for me, only the desire to discover what – word choice, title, structure – will work best.

The editors

Thank you both for your contributions.

4

"THE EXPO"

Guernica Magazine, March 15, 2013

Sybil Baker and Autumn Watts

This case study tackles both issues of fixing specific problems, and the give-and-take that occurs between author and editor to find a print-ready version which makes both happy without compromising the original aesthetic intentions beyond the author's baseline of tolerance. In broad terms, the issues encountered in Baker's "The Expo" fall into the categories of characterization, structure, and resolution, with a key focus on the relationship between the main characters and the "strange austerity" of the Shanghai landscape. We see Watts step in with specific suggestions for dealing with these. The approach is more hands-on than in other case studies. Ultimately, the editorial suggestions lead to a somewhat different story from that which is first submitted as a manuscript. In response to our questions, Baker and Watts reflect particularly on the revised ending – a process which was as much a push-and-pull between suggested changes and the original text as it was a full redraft. Baker's reflection that "revision often requires me to go deeper into their characters and not shy away from tension and conflict" is a pertinent reminder that much of the writing process happens in the rewriting, and draws attention to the fact that this can even be the first time the author really starts to appreciate the connections they have unconsciously embedded in the subtext.

When faced with producing a critical commentary on aspects of craft or process, it is not uncommon for student writers to insist that there was nothing conscious about the way in which their stories developed into a fully-fledged narrative, but this case study highlights how it is often *only* in the revision stage that we become fully aware of the imagery, metaphors, or conversely holes and inconsistencies in the story or plot. Far from being a frustrating additional hoop to jump through to see one's work in print, we can see that rigorous editing adds a vital, additional buffer to iron out any weaknesses that are hard to see from up close, a *second fix* to truly flesh a story out and embrace its potential. But this also introduces an element of rewriting that might make some uncomfortable. This case study asks quite defined questions of the revised edits, but equally it challenges the validity of certain decisions. We feel it is particularly useful for stimulating debate regarding the spectrum of editorial 'interference' and the obligation on the part of a writer to accept suggestions.

"The Expo"

They arrived when the sea was swelling, threatening to sweep the old world back with it. The rocky shore, barricaded by reeds sprouting from still pools of water, bordered an empty plaza with shiny monuments and statues, like a city of the future waiting for the new world to begin.

They were here for the World Expo in Shanghai, taking a long weekend, a rare holiday from their jobs, their first trip out of South Korea since they'd arrived four months ago. Laurie had wanted to go to Koh Samui in Thailand, where beaches stretched like linked arms circling, where she could pick a coconut freshly fallen and drink its milk with a straw. But Knox had already bought the plane tickets to Shanghai, and, before she'd had a chance to object, had booked a hotel through a travel agent in Itaewon. He'd wanted to go to the Expo since he was a kid, he confessed. The year he'd been born, 1982, the Expo had been held in Knoxville, and his parents had named him in honor of it, even though they lived in Johnson City. Her friends Aileen and Cilla were already in Koh Samui, getting high and meeting shirtless boys from around the world. But she had Knox, she reminded herself, and they didn't. Knox, who had saved her from disappearing. She felt sorry for people who did not have Knox in their lives, which meant she felt sorry for most of the world.

The airport taxi dropped them off at the end of a single lane road where a Holiday Inn Express, young and gleaming, awaited as if it had been built just for them. Workers sporting plastic nametags with English nicknames, like John and Meg and Amy, greeted them in Mandarin. Their room was almost-American, with cheerful phrases reminding guests that the free breakfast buffet was from 7:00 a.m. to 10:00 a.m. in the mornings and to please call the front desk if you needed a razor or toothbrush. They spent the first night enjoying the clean blandness of the room, the plumped pillows and flat screen TV, which yielded only one station in English, CCTV.

"It smells like a new Barbie," Laurie said, wistfully.

"It's like a post-apocalyptic 'Lady with a Lap Dog,'" Knox said. "A seaside with a plaza and a hotel."

"But there's no watermelon slice. No affair."

"Then maybe it's more like *The Sun Also Rises* or something by Joan Didion or Kundera."

"You mean it could be about anything," Laurie said. She had not read those books.

That evening on the empty plaza, Knox posed with two oversized statues of iron men, fishermen clad in bulky rubber boots, men seven feet tall, with barrel chests and thighs. A metal arch loomed over the bulk of the plaza, a gentle, open curve with beams that crisscrossed the clouds, like a large net dropped from the sky. They promenaded its length and at the other end discovered a concrete sculpture of an open book the size of their tiny bedroom in Seoul. The book sculpture opened to the middle, the pages filled with Chinese characters, with Laurie, Lilliputian-like, fitting in its crease. Except for the plaza and the sea, now receding, the world was landscaped grass and concrete, no trees or people, nothing else vertical except for the hotel, a lonely building, whether abandoned or waiting Laurie was not yet sure.

"This must be like Thailand," she said. She closed her eyes and pretended she was on a lounge chair with a book she could read, the sun warming her face.

"Better," Knox said, joining her in the crease of the book. "We're the only ones here."

The next morning they woke early, and in the darkness of the heavily draped room they had sex, lethargic and syrupy. After, wrapped in a towel damp from her shower, Laurie drew the drapes aside and admired the landscape, some stranger's unfinished dream. The only sound was Knox's slow, patient voice on the phone, asking the front desk for a razor, which he'd forgotten.

Outside the window, a tourist bus was chugging as a line of Chinese tourists in matching blue shirts and sun hats boarded. She thought about walking downstairs and joining them, taking the bus to wherever was next, more water or more trees or more people. But she could not disappear here, just as she could not disappear in Seoul, and before that, Tokyo. She'd disappeared for a while in San Francisco, just another thin blond girl with a leather jacket, and that had been good until it had not, when disappearing became not-existing, when she began to believe that she could become corners and tables and walls, that she could float above everything and everyone and not be noticed. Then Knox had found her one night at a party squatting in a dark space not far from the speakers, her usual spot for observation, and he'd joined her, narrating the events of the party as they unfolded as if she were blind and needed guidance. "See this guy," Knox had said, "he thinks he's Jay Gatsby or something, and this one, he looks like he's trapped in a Bret Easton Ellis novel – you know they used to wear skinny jeans in the eighties except they called them peg legs and they had zippers on the side." And on he went, for the rest of the night, until she finally asked him why he was talking to her like this. "Because I could tell you were about to disappear," he said. "I had to stop you."

Now, she heard him mutter into the receiver, "What skullduggery," then hang up the phone. Knox used words like that without irony. Scallywags. Shenanigans. She loved that about him. She felt his breath on her back as he circled her waist, allowing her towel to loosen. "Can I borrow your razor?" he whispered in her ear. "They don't understand English."

"Only if I can shave you."

"It's harder than it looks. I have a very angular face." But he allowed her – him sitting on the toilet, her bending over him, both of them naked, his face lathered (he had not forgotten the shaving cream), a warm wet towel around his neck because that's what Laurie remembered from the movies, and she shaved his face, whiskers collecting in the foam like black creatures caught in a blinding snow.

They dressed and arrived for breakfast at 8:30 a.m. Although the restaurant was empty, there was no place to sit. The tables towered with dirty dishes, spilt food, and half-finished plastic glasses of juice and tea. Chopsticks and forks were equally scattered. At one end of the room a woman pushed a cart, methodically cleaning each table, while a young man leaned against a wall, laconically watching the woman. They wore crisp uniforms and had English names affixed to their coats, yet they did not acknowledge Laurie or Knox.

"Are we ghosts?" Laurie whispered.

"You know, that's what they call white people. Or used to at least."

Laurie touched the smooth, pale hollow of Knox's cheek. "I can see why they'd think that."

The buffet table was almost barren. Rice porridge clung to the sides of one cooker, cracked balls of rice to another. A few hard-boiled eggs, peeled and soaked in soy sauce, were all that remained. Knox approached the man and pointed to the desecrated table and the sign above it, indicating that breakfast was until 10:00 a.m. The man shook his head and looked away. Laurie and Knox cleared a spot on one of the tables and ate their eggs while they watched the girl leisurely stack dirty plates in her cart at the other end of the room.

After breakfast, they discovered they were still an hour away from Shanghai, staying in a hotel in a city in China that did not yet officially exist. They saw into the future, the Chinese did, creating worlds Laurie could not even imagine, a future she felt privileged to glimpse. She was tired of the present – of her sad American life in Seoul. And so, when the hotel manager told them they must take a taxi to the bus station to get into Shanghai, she accepted the conditions willingly.

Knox did not see things her way. "Sounds like a lot of rigmarole. What if we don't get to see what we came for?"

"We will," Laurie said.

The taxi dropped them off at a provincial bus station in the middle of a field. They joined the line for Express Bus 4 as the hotel manager had instructed. After twenty minutes, a bus arrived and they boarded it. While Knox examined the subway map he'd picked up at the airport, Laurie looked out the window, waiting to catch a glimpse of Shanghai. For the first half hour the city was nowhere to be seen; instead they rambled by young growth forests, pastures, possibly farms, then closer in, tiny villages with tin roofs and chickens running about, rags hanging on tattered lines. Mud, outhouses, rusty spigots. Then, finally, they were in the city, and the bus dropped them off somewhere still far from the Expo, so they boarded the subway that would take them there according to Knox's map. After arriving at their chosen stop, they exited a subway station that faced a tourist information center. Banners announcing the arrival of the World Expo, in English and other languages, hung on the walls and from the ceiling of the almost empty office. One woman would not look up from her computer, clacking away on something seemingly important. A young man beside her slowly ate a banana, relishing every bite. Knox shuffled through the brochures stacked on a table near the door, hoping to find something in English. Laurie walked up to the man eating the banana, suddenly hungry. She waited for him to look at her, but he kept his eyes on the banana, which he carefully peeled a half inch after each bite. She was about to speak when she felt Knox's hand on her shoulder. He flashed a glossy brochure in front of her face. "We're closer than we thought."

By the time they arrived at the Expo, the lines to the entrance were wrapped around the metal rails like a snake sunning in the weak May light. They waited in line with the busloads of villagers who had descended on the complex. A family in front of them gnawed on small chicken wings extracted from a paper bag, sucking the bones dry then dropping them on the ground. Behind them, an older woman unfastened a small boy's flap in the front of his pants, allowing him to pee over the rails that guided them to the front. Knox kept his face buried in his brochure, unable to decide which country's exhibit he wanted to visit first. Laurie told him she wanted to go to Thailand.

Once inside, they were confronted with more lines winding and disappearing into the horizon. The longest line was for China, the largest pavilion in the complex, called The Crown of the East. Tourists sat on blankets and folding chairs, snacking from the feasts they'd brought in, umbrellas held overhead to shield them from the sun. Above them was taped a sign in black letters: Waiting Time About 8 Hours.

"Why would they spend all day waiting to see the country they live in?" Knox muttered.

"Because they want to see possibility," Laurie said. "That's why I'm going to Thailand."

They walked along the landscaped paths of the Expo, which were meticulously patterned with cushiony pink flowers that curved along a tiny concrete stream, until they arrived at Thailand's pavilion. A line like the others wrapped and looped with no apparent beginning or end. At the entrance stood two immense statue warriors, one green and one white, guarding the entrance. A clear pool of water surrounded the sides of the pavilion.

"Do we have to go inside? You get the idea," Knox said.

"I'm going in, I don't care how long it takes." She found the end of the line and prepared herself for the wait. "You don't have to," Laurie said. "I'll be okay."

He visored his face with his maps and sighed.

After two hours they entered an outdoor gallery surrounded by streams and fountains, screens of rainforests and manufactured lotus ponds. She walked through the Journey of Harmony, then A Harmony of Different tones, then A Harmony of Thais. She listened to music that sounded like women who were either very sad or very happy, then entered a temple and bowed in front of a green Buddha. In the last chamber, A Harmony of Thais, indigenous people draped her with heavy blankets dyed with berries and mountain flowers. At the exit was a bamboo hut café that smelled like the sea. Against the painted blue horizon, she drank coconut juice and ate a baby banana, tiny compared to the ones in the U.S. but still sweet and green, a little papery on her tongue.

When they emerged, Laurie said it was the best thing that had happened to her.

"It's not what I thought it would be," Knox said, as they dodged umbrella-wielding tourists protecting their skin from the fading sun. "But then, what ever is?"

They walked until they found a building with no line shared by small African countries like Mauritius and Eritrea and Gabon. They wandered the under-furnished stalls until it was late afternoon and time to find a way back to the hotel.

Knox had decided the best way back was to take the Shanghai Fastrapid, a magnetic levitation train, to the airport and then a taxi to the hotel from there. But when they arrived at the subway station, they discovered Fastrapid had closed an hour before, so they boarded the regular subway to the airport. Forty-five minutes later, still far from the airport, the subway stopped and shuttered its lights. An announcement blared through the speakers and everyone exited without complaint or resistance. Laurie and Knox emerged in an already darkened town and were suddenly swarmed by men desperate to take someone somewhere. Laurie extracted a card with the hotel's name and address on one side, a small map printed on the other, and waved it in the air. One of the men plucked the card and after glancing at the address, nodded, flashing his index and middle finger, indicating his price for the fare. They agreed on 200 renminbi, about thirty dollars, and climbed into his car, which, Laurie was quick to notice, had neither a cell phone on the dashboard nor a GPS system like the taxis in Seoul.

He drove at first with confidence, speeding away from the outskirts of the town, deeper into the forests and undeveloped land. Twice they narrowly averted accidents, when large carts powered by tiny motorcycle contraptions appeared suddenly from hidden curves in the unlit streets. After about half an hour, the taxi driver slowed down, leaning over his steering wheel, peering at roads as if searching for invisible signs or markers that would show him the way. He stopped at one intersection and asked a man pulling a cart, who at first gestured wildly, then shook his head. He drove them further down the road until all buildings disappeared and they were surrounded by trees, and then the man spoke in a loud anxious voice, holding three fingers up, wanting more money.

"No way," Knox said, shaking his head for emphasis.

"Just pay him," Laurie said in a low voice. She regretted she'd allowed Knox to keep the larger bills because, as he'd argued, she was forever losing things.

"We don't need him."

The driver resumed talking, pointing at the arrow on the gas gauge, which was dipping toward E. He held three fingers up, then four. Knox shook his head. Then the driver pulled over and turned the car off. Knox took out his Expo map and a ballpoint pen from his front shirt pocket and began scribbling. "I'm reporting you to the authorities, you scallywag," Knox said. The driver laughed, a sharp bark of one who has little to lose, and Laurie realized that the car was not his. She watched Knox write down what she read as gibberish, a code of numbers and letters she could not decipher. The driver continued laughing, beating his hand against the steering wheel. It was the laughing she could no longer take. Laurie opened the door.

Knox looked at her from inside the taxi. He was stooped, just a dark shadow from where she stood. "Get in," he pleaded. He reached for his wallet.

"Maybe he's the Misfit," Laurie said. "He wants us to stay in the car so he can kill us in some field because he doesn't believe in Jesus."

Knox shook his head. "It's just like this Paul Bowles story where this American is captured by some tribe in Morocco. They cut his tongue off, put him in a cage, and trot him around the desert."

The driver turned on the engine.

"Or maybe," she said, "it's like a large book that we can't read. Maybe this is the best moment of our lives, right now, even if we disappear."

She reached for Knox's hand and pulled him out of the car. She wrapped her arms around him, and Knox allowed the map he'd been clutching to fall to the pavement. The car sped away, leaving them alone in the dark.

They said nothing and began walking along the lampless road.

The editing of "The Expo"
by Sybil Baker
Edited by Autumn Watts

The following text is based on the original draft. Since the subsequent drafts contain additions and further changes, we have merged them together but without entirely changing the original. Some later additions and changes are highlighted in bold letters, as for instance some of the dialogue and the new ending. Unless we indicate something else in a footnote, all deleted text indicates Watts' line editing of the final draft. We display changes across different drafts to indicate the types of edits made in the process.

They arrived when the sea was swelling, threatening to sweep the old world back with it. The rocky shore, barricaded by reeds sprouting from still pools of water, bordered an empty plaza with shiny monuments and statues, like a city of the future waiting for the new world to begin.

They were here for the World Expo in Shanghai, taking a long weekend, a rare holiday from their jobs, their first trip out of South Korea since they'd arrived four months ago. Laurie had wanted to go to Koh Samui in Thailand, where beaches stretched like linked arms circling, where she could pick a coconut freshly fallen and drink its milk with a straw, where she and Knox would sleep in a straw hut and, because it was the rainy season, listen to the rain fall. But Knox had already bought the plane tickets to Shanghai, and, before she'd had a chance to object, had booked a hotel through a travel agent in Itaewon. He'd wanted to go the Expo since he was a kid, he confessed. The year he'd been born, 1982, the Expo had been held in Knoxville, and his parents had named him in honor of it, even though they lived in Johnson City. Before Knox, she'd only dated guys with names from Texas cities: Austin, Dallas, Houston. Her friends Aileen and Cilla were already in Koh Samui, getting high and meeting shirtless boys from around the world. But she had Knox, she reminded herself, and they didn't. Knox, who had saved her from disappearing. She felt sorry for people who did not have Knox in their lives, which meant she felt sorry for most of the world.

The airport taxi dropped them off at the end of a single lane road where a Holiday Inn Express, young and gleaming, awaited as if it had been built just for them. Workers sporting plastic name tags with English nicknames, like John and Meg and Amy, greeted them in Mandarin. Their room was almost-American, with cheerful phrases reminding guests that the free breakfast buffet was from seven to ten in the mornings, to please call the front desk if you needed a razor or toothbrush. They spent the first night enjoying the clean blandness of the room, the plumped pillows and flat screen TV which yielded only one station in English, CCTV.

"It smells like a new Barbie," Laurie said, wistfully.

"It's like a post-apocalyptic 'Lady with a Lap Dog,'" Knox said. "A seaside with a plaza and a hotel."

"But there's no watermelon slice, no affair."

"Then maybe it's more like *The Sun Also Rises* or something by Joan Didion or Kundera."

"You mean it could be about anything," Laurie said. She had not read those books.

That evening on the empty plaza, Knox posed with two oversized statues of iron men, fishermen clad in bulky rubber boots, men seven feet tall, with barrel chests and thighs, more Russian than Chinese. A metal arch loomed over the bulk of the plaza, a gentle open curve with beams that crisscrossed the clouds, like a large net dropped from the sky. They promenaded its length and at the other end discovered a concrete sculpture of an open book the size of their tiny bedroom in Seoul. The book sculpture opened to the middle, the pages filled with Chinese characters, with Laurie, Lilliputian-like, fitting in its crease. She did not know what the book said, but she didn't care, as she figured its secrets were beyond her. Except for the plaza and the sea, now receding, the visible world was landscaped grass and concrete, no trees or people, nothing else vertical except for the hotel, a lonely building, whether abandoned or waiting Laurie was not yet sure.

The next morning they woke early, and in the darkness of the heavily draped room they had sex, lethargic and syrupy. After, wrapped in a towel damp from her shower, Laurie drew the drapes aside and admired the landscape, some stranger's unfinished dream. The only sound was Knox's slow, patient voice on the phone, asking the front desk for a razor, which he'd forgotten.

Outside the window, a tourist bus was chugging as a line of Chinese tourists in matching blue shirts and sun hats boarded. She thought about walking downstairs and joining them, taking the bus to wherever was next, more water or more trees or more people, and wherever she was she'd look up at the sky and try to count stars. But she was a white girl. She could not disappear here, just as she could not disappear in Seoul, and before that, Tokyo. She'd disappeared for a while in San Francisco, just another thin blond girl with a leather jacket, and that had been good until it had not, when disappearing became not-existing, when she began to believe that she could become corners and tables and walls, that she could float above everything and everyone and not be noticed. Then Knox had found her one night at a party squatting in a dark space not far from the speakers, her usual spot for observation, and he'd joined her, narrating the events of the party as they unfolded as if she were blind and needed guidance. "See this guy," Knox had said, "he thinks he's Jay Gatsby or something, and this one, he looks like he's trapped in a Brett Easton Ellis novel – you know they used to wear skinny jeans in the eighties except they called them peg legs and they had zippers on the side. ~~My mom used to wear them.~~" And on he went, for the rest of the night, until she finally asked him why he was talking to her like this. "Because I could tell you were about to disappear," he said. "I had to stop you."

Now, she heard him mutter into the receiver, "What skullduggery," then hanging up the phone. Knox used words like that without irony. Scallywags. Shenanigans. She loved that about him. She felt his breath on her back as he circled her waist, allowing her towel to loosen. "Can I borrow your razor?" he whispered in her ear. "They don't understand English."

"Only if I can shave you."

"It's harder than it looks. I have a very angular face." But he allowed her, him sitting on the toilet, her bending over him, both of them naked, his face lathered (he had not forgotten the shaving cream), a warm wet towel around his neck because that's what Laurie remembered from the movies, and she shaved his face, whiskers collecting in the foam like black creatures caught in a blinding snow.

They dressed and arrived for breakfast at 8:30 a.m. Although the restaurant was empty, there was no place to sit. The tables towered with dirty dishes, spilt food, half-finished plastic glasses of juice and tea. Chopsticks and forks were equally scattered. At one end of the room a woman pushed a cart, methodically cleaning each table, while a young man leaned against a wall, laconically watching the woman. They wore crisp uniforms and had English names affixed to their coats, yet they did not acknowledge Laurie or Knox.

"Are we ghosts?" Laurie whispered.

"You know, that's what they call white people. Or used to at least."

The buffet table was almost barren. Rice porridge clung to the sides of one cooker, cracked balls of rice to another. A few hard-boiled eggs, peeled and soaked in soy sauce, were all that remained. Knox approached the man and pointed to the desecrated table and the sign above it, indicating that breakfast was until ten. The man shook his head and looked away. They cleared a spot on one of the tables and ate their eggs while they watched the girl leisurely stack dirty plates in her cart at the other end of the room.

After breakfast they discovered they were still an hour away from Shanghai, staying in a hotel in a city in China that did not yet officially exist. They saw into the future, the Chinese did, creating worlds Laurie could not even imagine, a future she felt privileged to glimpse. She was tired of the present, of her sad American life in Seoul. And so, when the hotel manager told them they must take a taxi to the bus station to get into Shanghai, she accepted the conditions willingly.~~, for what other American had been given this gift to see the future.~~

Knox did not see things her way. ~~"That travel agent really fucked us over," he said. "She told me it was a good location. We're in the middle of nowhere! She's obviously in cahoots with these guys."~~ "Sounds like a lot of rigmarole. What if we don't get to see what we came for?"

"We will," Laurie said.[1]

The taxi dropped them off at a provincial bus station in the middle of a field. They joined the line for Express Bus 4 as the hotel manager had instructed. After twenty minutes a bus arrived and they boarded it. While Knox examined the subway map he'd picked up at the airport, Laurie looked out the window, waiting to catch a glimpse of Shanghai. For the first half hour the city was nowhere to be seen; instead they rambled by young growth forests, pastures, possible farms, then closer in, tiny villages with tin roofs and chickens running about, rags hanging on tattered lines. Mud, outhouses, rusty spigots. Then, finally, they were in the city, and the bus dropped them off somewhere still far from the Expo, so they boarded the subway that would take them there according to Knox's map. After arriving at their chosen stop, they exited a subway station which faced a tourist information center~~, its sign in large English letters~~. On the walls and from the ceiling of the almost empty office hung banners in English and other languages announcing the arrival of the World Expo. One woman would not look up from her computer, clacking away on something seemingly important. A young man beside her slowly ate a banana, relishing every bite. Knox shuffled through the brochures stacked on a table near the door, hoping to find something in English. ~~He finally found a glossy brochure with a map to the Expo, its entrance only a few blocks away. They left without ever being acknowledged, and Laura wondered if perhaps they were ghosts after all.~~ **Laurie walked up to the man eating the banana, suddenly hungry. She waited for him to look at her, but he kept his eyes on the banana, which he carefully peeled a half inch after each bite. She was about to speak when she felt Knox's hand on her shoulder. He flashed a glossy brochure in front of her face, ~~so that she could no longer see the banana guy.~~ "We don't need him," he said. "We're closer than we thought."**

By the time they arrived, the lines to the entrance were wrapped around the metal rails like a snake sunning in the weak May sun. They waited in line with the busloads of ~~Chinese~~ villagers who had descended on the complex. A family in front of them gnawed on small chicken wings extracted from a paper bag, ~~smacking loudly with happiness,~~ sucking the bones dry then dropping them on the ground. Behind them, an older woman unfastened a small boy's flap in the front of his pants, allowing him to pee over the rails that guided them to the front. Knox kept his face buried in his brochure, unable to decide which country he wanted to visit first.

---

1 Cut and changed by Baker.

Once inside, they were confronted with more lines winding and disappearing into the horizon. The longest line was for China, the largest pavilion in the complex, called The Crown of the East. Tourists sat on blankets and folding chairs, snacking from the feasts of food they'd brought in, umbrellas held overhead to shield them from the sun. Above them was taped a sign in black letters: Waiting Time About 8 Hours.

"Why would they spend all day waiting to see the country they live in?" Knox muttered.

"Because they want to see possibility," Laurie said.

~~Instead of joining one of the lines which waited for countries they'd already seen, they chose to walk along the landscaped paths of the complex, which was meticulously patterned with cushiony pink flowers that curved along a tiny concrete stream. Finally at the end of the complex, they found a building with no line shared by small African countries like Mauritius and Eritrea and Gabon. They wandered the under-furnished stalls until it was late afternoon and time to find a way back to the hotel.~~[2]

They walked along the landscaped paths of the complex, which was meticulously patterned with cushiony pink flowers that curved along a tiny concrete stream until they arrived at Thailand's pavilion. A line like the others wrapped and looped with no apparent beginning or end. At the entrance stood two immense statue warriors, one green and one white, guarding the entrance. A clear pool of water surrounded the sides of the pavilion.

~~**"It's even better than I dreamed," Laurie said.**~~

"Do we have to go inside? You get the idea," Knox said.

"I'm going in, I don't care how long it takes." She found the end of the line and prepared herself for the wait. ~~**Knox shifted from one foot to the next.**~~ **"You don't have to," Laurie said. "I'll be okay."**

He visored his face with his maps and sighed.

They waited in line for two hours before they entered Thailand. She walked through the Journey of Harmony, then A Harmony of Different tones, than A Harmony of Thais. She listened to music that sounded like women who were either very sad or very happy. She entered a temple and bowed in front of a green Buddha. She met mountain people and watched them weave colored blankets dyed with berries and flowers. At the beach, she drank coconut juice and ate a baby banana, tiny compared to the ones in the US, but still sweet and green, a little papery on her tongue.[3]

---

2   Cut by Baker during revision.
3   Watts commented on this revision: "I'm a little confused about the scale here, especially the beach. Can you clarify the environment a little bit more?" The final version can be seen in the published story.

When they emerged, Laurie said it was the best thing that had happened to her.

"It's not what I thought it would be," Knox said, as they dodged umbrella-wielding tourists protecting their skin from the fading sun. "But then, what ever is?"

They walked until they found a building with no line shared by small African countries like Mauritius and Eritrea and Gabon. They wandered the under-furnished stalls until it was late afternoon and time to find a way back to the hotel.

Knox had decided the best way back was to take the Shanghai Fastrapid, a magnetic levitation train, to the airport and then a taxi to the hotel from there. But when they arrived at the subway station, they discovered Fastrapid had closed an hour ago, so they boarded the regular subway to the airport. Forty-five minutes later, still far from the airport, the subway stopped and shuttered its lights. An announcement blared through the speakers and everyone exited without complaint or resistance. Laurie and Knox emerged in an already darkened town and were suddenly swarmed by men desperate to take someone somewhere. Laurie extracted a card with the hotel's name and address on one side, a small map printed on the other, and waved it in the air. One of the men plucked the card and after glancing at the address, nodded, flashing his index and middle finger, indicating his price for the fare. They agreed on 200 renminbi, about 30 dollars, and climbed into his car, which, Laurie was quick to notice, had neither a cell phone on the dashboard nor a GPS system like the taxis in Seoul.

He drove at first with confidence, speeding away from the outskirts of the town, deeper into the forests and undeveloped land. Twice they narrowly averted accidents, when large carts powered by tiny motorcycle contraptions appeared suddenly from hidden curves in the unlit streets. After about half an hour, the taxi driver slowed down, leaning over his steering wheel, peering at roads as if searching for invisible signs or markers that would show him the way. He stopped at one intersection and asked a man pulling a cart, who at first gestured wildly, then shook his head. He drove them further down the road until all buildings disappeared and they were surrounded by trees, and then the man spoke in a loud anxious voice, holding three fingers up, wanting more **money**.

"No way," Knox said, shaking his head for emphasis.

"Knox, just pay him," Laurie said in a low voice. ~~She regretted she'd allowed Knox to be the keeper of all their cash and could not pay the driver herself.~~ **She regretted she'd allowed Knox to keep the larger bills because, as he'd argued, she was forever losing things.**

~~"I hate getting ripped off," he said. "We'll wait him out."~~

"We don't need him."[4]

The driver resumed talking, pointing at the arrow on the gas gauge, which was dipping toward E. He held three fingers up, then four. Knox shook his head. Then

---

4   Changed by Baker in the subsequent drafts.

the driver pulled over and turned the car off. Knox took out his Expo map and a ballpoint pen from his front shirt pocket and began scribbling. "I'm reporting you to the authorities, you scallywag," Knox said. The driver laughed, a sharp bark of one who has little to lose, and Laurie realized that the car was not his. She watched Knox continue to write down what she read as gibberish, a code of numbers and letters she could not decipher. The driver continued laughing, beating his hand against the steering wheel. Laurie opened the door~~., and Knox followed her out. The car sped away leaving them alone on the dark.~~

~~They said nothing, and began walking along the lampless road, wondering if someone would find them, wondering if they wanted to be found. Then Knox stopped and allowed the map he'd been clutching to fall on the road. He looked up at the sky, as if he were hoping the stars would guide him.~~

~~"It's just like this Paul Bowles story where this American is captured by some tribe in Morocco," Knox finally said. "They cut his tongue off, put him in a cage, and trot him around the desert. Or maybe it's more like 'A Good Man is Hard to Find.' The Misfit could be in these very woods."~~

~~Laurie wrapped her arms around him from behind, resting her head on his back. "It's okay Knox, that's not our story." She breathed into his bones. "Our story hasn't been written yet, it's not like any other, it's not the future we anticipated, and that's a good thing. In fact this is the best moment of our lives, right now, and we'll never get it back, this moment, when, even if for the length of our breaths or a lifetime, we truly disappear."~~

Knox looked at her from inside the taxi. He was stooped, just a dark shadow from where she stood. "Get in," he pleaded. He reached for his wallet.

"Maybe he's the Misfit," Laurie said. "He wants us to stay in the car so he can kill us in some field because he doesn't believe in Jesus."

He shook his head, his eyes bright and trembling. "It's just like this Paul Bowles story where this American is captured by some tribe in Morocco. They cut his tongue off, put him in a cage, and trot him around the desert."

The driver turned on the engine.

"Or maybe," she said, "it's like a large book that we can't read. Maybe this is the best moment of our lives, right now, even if we disappear."

She reached for Knox's hand and pulled him out of the car. She wrapped her arms around him, and Knox allowed the map he'd been clutching to fall to the ~~road~~ pavement.[5] The car sped away leaving them alone in the dark.

They said nothing, and began walking along the lampless road.

---

5   Watts changed "road" to "pavement" after Baker added the new ending to avoid the repetition.

"The Expo"
Conversation with Sybil Baker and Autumn Watts

The editors

Sybil, tell us briefly about this story, and what were the main issues Autumn Watts, your editor at *Guernica*, wanted you to work on?

Baker

Many of my short stories start with an image or a small event that I see or experience that allows fictional possibilities of discovery. Often this means taking something ordinary and then asking "what if?""The Expo" came from such a place. My husband and I, while visiting friends in Korea, decided to take a long weekend trip to Shanghai and the World Expo. We ended up booking a hotel very similar to the one in the story, and on our way home from The Expo our taxi driver couldn't find our hotel, which was in a remote place. He wanted more money from us, and my husband, feeling that we were being ripped off, refused. I remember feeling afraid in the taxi, realizing suddenly how vulnerable we were, not speaking the language in the countryside where we had no ability to contact anyone. We eventually made it back to the hotel without incident, but I wondered, what if the taxi driver had decided to drop us off in the middle of nowhere, or worse, to rob us or do something even more heinous? The story began with that idea, but the actual incidents in the story and the couple were fictional. In an early draft of the story, I opened with a sentence echoing the first sentence from Flannery O'Connor's "A Good Man Is Hard to Find," which is referenced in "The Expo:""She didn't want to go to Shanghai." While that sentence disappeared from subsequent drafts, it was a way for me to establish the conflict between Laurie and Knox and opened the possibility for me to use some literary references in the story.

Autumn Watts pointed out some obvious deficiencies in the story, mostly that the relationship between Knox and Laurie was not that balanced, that Laurie was too passive, allowing Knox too much power. Once Watts pointed that out, I could easily see this as a problem and rewrote the story focusing on Knox and Laurie's relationship more. I also paid more attention to the story's structure, trying to escalate the obstacles to each character's opposing desires. I added a scene where Laurie decides to go into the Thai Pavilion and Knox follows, reversing the power structure of the relationship at the midpoint of the story. I revised the ending to reflect the tension of their relationship.

With Watts' edits, we ended on an image of the lampless road instead of dialogue. By changing Laurie's and Knox's exchange of literary examples before Knox gets out of the taxi, the ending shifts to Knox giving in to Laurie, reflecting the power shift in the story. The last image shows them together, without the map Knox realizes is useless. I also wanted the ending to echo the beginning, with Knox and Laurie leaving the old world behind, and walking down the unknown, new world.

Besides copy editing, I find that revision often requires me to go deeper into their characters and not shy away from tension and conflict. In this case, Autumn's editorial suggestions helped shape the story's structure and illuminate the tension between the couple which had not been explored in earlier drafts.

The editors

In your correspondence, Watts writes:

> I love the strange austerity of the landscape and Laurie's yearning response to it. Her relationship with Knox drives the heart of the story, but I'd like it to be even more substantial and complex. Laurie is passive until the very end, following Knox without complaint even when he's selfish or irritating. I do love how their trip disintegrates until they wind up lost and walking down a dark road, and she finally interrupts Knox's insistence on narrating their life through other stories, but as it stands I need the ending to have more grip, perhaps by illuminating the building tensions in their relationship? I'd love to see a bit more texture to Laurie. The end seems to resolve too much, too easily.

It is clear that the editor finds the story compelling enough as it is, but at same time wants to see what some particular changes would do to this story. Watts' suggestion seems to imply two things, both that the story is complete and working well, and that it requires what some might consider a larger change since it concerns characterization. This may not entail major rewrites, but ultimately, since this is a character-driven narrative, the editorial suggestion leads to a somewhat different story. Can you say something more about this particular issue with regards to "The Expo" but also in general, in terms of editorial practices as such? How common is it, from your experience, for an editor to ask for changes in the characters?

Baker

One of my own issues as a writer is that I often don't push my main characters far enough – that is, I keep them too passive. When I have worked with editors on revisions, this has been one aspect that I have gladly revised. In that sense, I don't know if I am changing the character as much as giving her more agency and allowing her an arc, rather than keeping her more passive and static. With all of the editors I've worked with (including on my novels), I have felt that their suggestions were in service of the story. The changes are ultimately my own, and up to me to determine the way that I will make a character more active.

Watts

I fell in love with this story the first time I read it, but I felt some aspects still had room to grow. In these situations, I like to reach out to the author and elicit their thoughts and their willingness to explore those possibilities. Sometimes I think there are places where the story might reach a little more or hold back a little more, and "The Expo" was a great example of both. As Sybil points out, her revisions gave her character more agency and arc without changing the heart of the character or the story. Editing is a subjective process that can also just come down to the taste of the editor, and I'm conscious of that. Ideally, I aim to help a writer clarify, uncover or solidify their intentions in the story, but I'm open to argument, too, and I like to see where the writer's instincts lead the revision.

The editors

Watts suggests the ending needs some work, and there is a hint at what is weaker in the first version and in which direction it should go. This is ultimately tied to the issue of characterization. The new ending would come out of those revisions in the dynamics. The image of the lampless road changes the drive of the story, the locus of it in some ways, which almost retrofits a theme or a meaning to the story – it becomes more about the tension and imbalance in the relationship. Sybil, were you resistant to changing the ending? When you received the suggestions, did you feel that Watts' point about the ending was clear enough, or did you initially want more guidelines? Watts does not suggest any particular solutions. Have you ever worked with an editor who made particular suggestions about the content, specific things they wanted to see? Below are the original and the final endings:

The Original Ending

"I'm reporting you to the authorities, you scallywag," Knox said. The driver laughed, a sharp bark of one who has little to lose, and Laurie realized that the car was not his. She watched Knox continue to write down what she read as gibberish, a code of numbers and letters she could not decipher. The driver continued laughing, beating his hand against the steering wheel. Laurie opened the door, and Knox followed her out. The car sped away leaving them alone on the dark.

They said nothing, and began walking along the lampless road, wondering if someone would find them, wondering if they wanted to be found. Then Knox stopped and allowed the map he'd been clutching to fall on the road. He looked up at the sky, as if he were hoping the stars would guide him.

"It's just like this Paul Bowles story where this American is captured by some tribe in Morocco," Knox finally said. "They cut his tongue off, put him in a cage, and trot him around the desert. Or maybe it's more like 'A Good Man is Hard to Find.' The Misfit could be in these very woods."

Laurie wrapped her arms around him from behind, resting her head on his back. "It's okay Knox, that's not our story." She breathed into his bones. "Our story hasn't been written yet, it's not like any other, it's not the future we anticipated, and that's a good thing. In fact this is the best moment of our lives, right now, and we'll never get it back, this moment, when, even if for the length of our breaths or a lifetime, we truly disappear."

Knox looked at her from inside the taxi. He was stooped, just a dark shadow from where she stood. "Get in," he pleaded. He reached for his wallet.

"Maybe he's the Misfit," Laurie said. "He wants us to stay in the car so he can kill us in some field because he doesn't believe in Jesus."

Final Ending

Knox looked at her from inside the taxi. He was stooped, just a dark shadow from where she stood. "Get in," he pleaded. He reached for his wallet.

"Maybe he's the Misfit," Laurie said. "He wants us to stay in the car so he can kill us in some field because he doesn't believe in Jesus."

Knox shook his head. "It's just like this Paul Bowles story where this American is captured by some tribe in Morocco. They cut his tongue off, put him in a cage, and trot him around the desert."

The driver turned on the engine.

"Or maybe," she said, "it's like a large book that we can't read. Maybe this is the best moment of our lives, right now, even if we disappear."

She reached for Knox's hand and pulled him out of the car. She wrapped her arms around him, and Knox allowed the map he'd been clutching to fall to the pavement. The car sped away, leaving them alone in the dark.

They said nothing and began walking along the lampless road.

Baker

I often have problems with endings, and they take several revisions to land in the right place. In my experience, an editor helps point out parts of a story that I may not see, to provide that "lamp" in a lampless road. Writing is a process of a discovery. A good editor helps me discover what the best of this story can be. In that sense, I am usually open to revising a piece, and welcome it, if I trust the editor, which in this case I did. I go in with the attitude that the editor is working with me to make the piece better.

Watts

My feeling about the original ending was that it over-explained and tidied up too neatly. I suggested ending the story earlier because for Laurie, that act of bringing Knox out of the car had so much power and really punctuated the shift in their relationship that Sybil wanted to highlight. However, my first impulse with where to end the story left it in a fairly stark place, which Sybil had also mentioned she was trying to avoid. I generally don't like suggesting specific solutions about content, because I do believe it interferes with the writer's intuition, and of course it's not my story. I think the editor can serve as more of a mirror or a flag to whatever feels off, and I trust that the author will discover how best to improve with results that please and surprise us both. In the end, I really loved how Sybil unpacked that scene and restrained it at the same time. The image of them alone in the dark, walking along the lampless road, was just so much more vast and suggestive than the dialogue-heavy original.

The editors

We wonder about the lines put back into the narrative. Autumn, you pared down the ending for dramatic effect but then added some older lines Sybil had cut. Was she over-editing herself and did you want to push her back to the original version? Why did it make more sense to revert to the older version? We find that it shows how organic the entire process is. What seems wrong at one point can become relevant again and the craft of the editor shows this in some form of multidirectional vision.

Watts

I find that after revision, lines that didn't ring quite right can take on a different resonance. Editing and writing are not linear processes. There's much back and forth and circling around, interrogating and revisiting. Sometimes what I'm asking for an author to do is experiment: to try something out and see what settles into place. Sybil's revision shifted the center of gravity in the ending and rebalanced lines that hadn't really worked as well before. Without Laurie's longer speech at the end, the bit about the Misfit – which was originally said by Knox, but then switched to Laurie in the revision – had a lightness now against Knox's fearful rigidity, underscoring Laurie's empowerment and her compassion for him.

The editors

Let us look at some specific cuts, additions, and changes of content. Can you say something about each, how they affect characterization and the story as such? These are some of the cuts we are interested in:

> Laurie had wanted to go to Koh Samui in Thailand, where beaches stretched like linked arms circling, where she could pick a coconut freshly fallen and drink its milk with a straw, where she and Knox would sleep in a straw hut and, because it was the rainy season, listen to the rain fall.
>
> The year he'd been born, 1982, the Expo had been held in Knoxville, and his parents had named him in honor of it, even though they lived in Johnson City. Before Knox, she'd only dated guys with names from Texas cities: Austin, Dallas, Houston.
>
> She thought about walking downstairs and joining them, taking the bus to wherever was next, more water or more trees or more people, and wherever she was she'd look up at the sky and try to count stars. But she was a white girl. She could not disappear here, just as she could not disappear in Seoul, and before that, Tokyo.

And so, when the hotel manager told them they must take a taxi to the bus station to get into Shanghai, she accepted the conditions willingly.~~, for what other American had been given this gift to see the future?~~

He flashed a glossy brochure in front of her face.~~, so that she could no longer see the banana guy. "We don't need him," he said.~~ "We're closer than we thought."

Watts

Most of the cuts I suggested were to help tighten the pace in places where the writing slowed down for me or seemed over-described. As for Sybil's changes in content, I think the second reference to ghosts really just pointed out a tension that was already communicated through more subtle cues, as displacement and unease simply vibrate throughout that whole scene. When Sybil added the line where Laurie touches Knox's cheek, I think it brought energy and layers to Laurie's character, which had been both more passive and less complex in the earlier version.

The editors

This section concerns the change of content:

> **First draft:** A young man beside her slowly ate a banana, relishing every bite. Knox shuffled through the brochures stacked on a table near the door, hoping to find something in English. He finally found a glossy brochure with a map to the Expo, its entrance only a few blocks away. They left without ever being acknowledged, and Laura wondered if perhaps they were ghosts after all.

> **Final draft:** Laurie walked up to the man eating the banana, suddenly hungry. She waited for him to look at her, but he kept his eyes on the banana, which he carefully peeled a half inch after each bite. She was about to speak when she felt Knox's hand on her shoulder. He flashed a glossy brochure in front of her face. "We're closer than we thought."

In this case, we wonder why the line that specifically brings back the image of them being ghosts, that post-colonial unease that Laurie has and Knox seems less sensitive to, has been removed. It is the line that foregrounds their displacement, their invisibility, that they are unacknowledged. This may be where the story begins to change direction from original to final draft.

Baker

For me the first part focuses on outside action and little action from Laurie, except her wondering about being ghosts. In the second, Laurie's "hunger" suggests that she wants something she doesn't have – yet. That she is going to speak but Knox stops her does highlight the dynamic of their relationship, and as you suggest, hints at the power change that will continue in the story.

The editors

How about the change of content in this section?

> **First draft:**
> Knox did not see things her way.
>   "That travel agent really fucked us over," he said. "She told me it was a good location. We're in the middle of nowhere! She's obviously in cahoots with these guys."

> **Final draft:**
> Knox did not see things her way. "Sounds like a lot of rigmarole. What if we don't get to see what we came for?"
>   "We will," Laurie said.

Baker

The second one develops Knox's character as one who uses old-fashioned words (in this case by changing "fucked over" to "rigmarole"). Also by him asking a question which Laurie answers, which continues to develop their own relationship.

The editors

We wonder about this addition:

> "Are we ghosts?" Laurie whispered.
>   "You know, that's what they call white people. Or used to at least."
>   **Laurie touched the smooth, pale hollow of Knox's cheek. "I can see why they'd think that."**

Baker

This again brings the scene and action back to Laurie instead of keeping her passive – she strokes Knox's cheek and answers his question. She has some understanding or empathy for how people might perceive them, opening up possibilities for her.

The editors

Thank you both for your contribution.

5

"THE KING OF THE BALL"

Two Thirds North, 2016

Friðrik Sólnes Jónsson, Lucy Durneen,
Adnan Mahmutović and Anna Crofts

Friðrik Sólnes Jónsson submitted "The King of the Ball" to *Two Thirds North* in autumn 2015 and it was selected for publication in the 2016 issue. The first edit was done by Lucy Durneen, followed by Adnan Mahmutović. The assistant editor Anna Crofts, who championed the story throughout the selection process, was involved in the final stages of the editing process.

This particular case raises a number of issues related to both the process of editing and the character of the relationship(s) in the process. One important segment, that of content, called for an involvement of several editors, none of which had complete authority over the process. It is not unusual for editors to cut the so-called 'fat', the excess of information that can have a negative effect on the narrative flow. In fact, cutting is perhaps the core of editing as such. There are many famous cases, such as Carver-Lish and Perkins-Wolfe. In the case of "The King of the Ball", Durneen made a few cuts following her editorial instinct that the information did not add to the narrative and looked excessive. The second editor, Mahmutović, who was supposed to give the story one final touch, agreed and offered minimal edits, but the assistant editor Anna Crofts, who was the one responsible for the acceptance of the story, noted that the missing content caused certain issues necessary both for characterization and storyline. Mahmutović discussed this with Sólnes Jónsson, after which the information was brought back into the story, but rewritten. This particularity in the editing process is going to be core of the discussion between Mahmutović, Durneen, and Sólnes Jónsson at the end of this chapter, but it is important to highlight the idea that sometimes editing can be "adding" or "retrieving" of that which was lost in the editing, perhaps the way we speak about something being lost in translation. This is similar to Angela Redman's discussion of carvers pre-Lish drafts, which contain information essential for adding certain depth to the characters. In that case, what was lost-in-edit (content) helped create something gained-in-edit (style). The "retrieval" was, of course, not simple. It involved a consideration of what made Durneen cut it in the first place. It was a matter of identifying the real issue in those passages which then allowed for reinsertion of content and further rewriting.

The case of Sólnes Jónsson shows not only the possibility of editing-as-retrieval, but also how several editors can work in symbiosis towards the final goal. Surely, it does not allow for, or in fact it prevents the making of a stereotyped antagonistic relationship between authors and editors.

Below follow: the published story, the draft with the edits and a conversation about the process.

"The King of the Ball"

In the small town of Akureyri in Iceland, the sixties didn't arrive until we were already halfway into the seventies. What's more, not much of the revolutionary spirit of the sixties made it through intact. Only some music and hairstyles. My generation's parents belonged to the old system of farmers and fishermen who moved to the town from the rural areas and still remembered having to use an outhouse or a bedpan and not having electricity. Or so were we told, over and over, through our childhoods. We were therefore genuinely grateful for all the modern comforts and wouldn't even think of making a fuss over things like social stratification or the Viet Nam war. People who are grateful like that tend to be quite conservative.

As the truism would have it, people grew up faster back then. Looking at my old class photo from when we graduated from tenth grade, everyone seemed really grown up. The men looked like proper adults, most in dark brown or black suits, some with sideburns, some even with full beards, even if they were only 16 or 17. The teacher was sitting a little to the left of the group. He had large black-rimmed glasses and looked a lot like Carlos the Jackal.

At school, agents, spokespersons or delegates from different organizations or companies had full access to students during school hours. These visits were heartily welcomed by teachers and students alike since the normal curriculum was often repetitive and dull. In the space of a single school year our class would be given over to all sorts of delegates and officials on a regular basis. Someone from the Gideons International would hand out copies of the New Testament and say a few words about the benefits of letting Jesus Christ into our lives. A man from the Independence Party warned against the devastating effect on our frail economy if taxes or wages would be raised. Númi Þorkell from the YMCA hunted for volunteers both for the nearby lakeside boys' summer camp as well as the mission in Kenya.

The most memorable visit was an emissary from the Good Templars, which was quite a formidable organization in our town. This small and jittery man was around 60 and had a frown on his face like a mouse looking upwards to sniff at something. He played us a short silent movie using the school's huge projector and every now and then described to us what was happening on the screen in short agitated bursts of speech. The film was Scandinavian, titled "Balkongen," or, as the man translated it, "The King of the Ball." In our dialect, the word "ball" wasn't just used for formal dances but for any type of get-togethers with music and drinks. The film showed a house party in an apartment block with people drinking, playing records and a few dancing in a clunky way. The film seemed to have a lot of dialogue but our narrator waited patiently through those with his hands crossed over his groin. He sprang into motion when a dark haired man entered the frame. "There he is! The King of the Ball!" He tapped the textile projector screen hard with his finger, denting the picture. "Look at him! He's totally deranged from drink. You'll see where that gets you."

The King of the Ball was a normal looking fellow in a light-colored suit. He had a drink in his hand and smiled a lot but he didn't participate in any of the dialogues and was mostly seen in the background or in panoramic shots of the party. The short film reached its tragic crescendo during a scene where two women had a heated argument which lead to one of them falling off the balcony. The old Templar guy tapped on the poor woman who was lying on the pavement below. She raised her head slightly to look up towards the balcony and some terrified guests before falling back down lifeless, dramatically succumbing to her injuries. "This is what you get when you consort with the King of the Ball!"

But the King of the Ball hadn't been on screen in a while and he wasn't seen again until the guests were all filing out of the building, looking sombre and miserable. The Templar gave the screen a slightly softer tap this time.

"He must be really happy with himself now, the king."

Credits rolled.

After a dramatic pause the old man waxed poetic and asked us to think about the hundreds of seeds that would never become flowers because of the King of the Ball and others of his ilk. Then he thanked the teacher, said his goodbyes and disappeared with his two huge reels of film in their metal casings. His message was mostly lost on us. The film was more confusing than inspiring but I think most of the boys in class that day where left harboring a secret wish to some day become the King of the Ball.

The years after I finished the tenth grade went by quickly. I started going out to sea with my father who was the captain on a fishing trawler. I had been going every now and then during summers since I was ten, more to spend time with my father than to do work, but the crew were quick to find uses for me so I mostly ran around with the ship's dog, Lárpera, sharpened knives, helped mend the nets, or delivered messages. Spending time with my father was also nice. He was almost always out at sea and when he came home the atmosphere was tense and he mostly wanted to be left alone in his study. The first time he was home at Christmas I was already thirteen and it felt strange to see someone else sitting in my mother's chair.

After the tenth grade, I was out at sea so much I missed out on countless parties, camping trips and friends' weddings. I also missed out on the not-yet-so-famous Kinks playing in our local movie theater, and Led Zeppelin, playing in our giant handball arena at the peak of their career. It was perhaps no big surprise then that the King of the Ball loomed large in my thoughts during this time.

A chance presented itself when the crew was in the small harbor city of Hull with a few days' shore leave. The plan was to leave the old trawler to be scrapped and then sail home on a brand new one. My father was busy with moving equipment between the two trawlers and the rest of the crew would visit prostitutes and get anchors tattooed on their forearms marking the occasion, with "Hull 1974" inscribed beneath. The first thing I did was to get on the next train to London. At Piccadilly Circus I walked straight into Aquascutum, which sold high quality clothes for gentlemen, and proceeded to dress myself up like a king. I bought a suit and an overcoat and some dress shirts, shoes, leather gloves, a belt, and a scarf. It cost around two months' wages but I didn't care. I was always working and I never had a chance to spend anything. A week later we were docking again back home. Akureyri had never seemed smaller and the mountains around it had never seemed bigger and more imposing. Seeing the dockworkers and the old cars parked nearby made me feel like I had just traveled back in time.

As I walked back home over the gravel lot with the taxis I could see posters advertising a ball that very evening, with a band playing and everything. This was my chance. I got dressed in my new clothes and drove to the ball. I sat in my car for a while close to the venue, our handball arena, and listened to the national radio. Sailors' Requests was on, mostly playing upbeat accordion music. I took swigs from a small vodka bottle and smoked Royale cigarettes. I had grown quite tall and the roof of my Volkswagen beetle flattened the top of my Afro hairdo. When I'd polished off the vodka I got out and walked towards the arena.

It was the time of year which our poet Halldór Laxness had described as the time between hay and grass, when winter was supposed to be over but spring was not in sight, and men and animals used to drop like flies. This was in the olden days, which in Iceland lasted until WWII, when the blessed war made everyone rich and modern.

The air was cold and crisp and after six weeks of diesel fumes I felt I could smell the oxygen in the air. The cold didn't come with the wind but rather seemed to radiate from the ground and the yellow grass was frozen so it made a soft creaking sound when you walked on it. There was already a line outside the venue. Most of the people were dressed up but a few of the men seemed to have just headed there straight after work. They looked like the dockworkers I'd seen earlier – in dirty and worn woolen sweaters with sixpence caps and specks of coarse snuff tobacco around their noses and mouths – and they made me feel the sort of confidence that's born out of sheer contempt for one's fellow man. I was also drunk and looking like a goddamned prince. I walked past the line and went straight inside. I didn't even stop to pay for a ticket. I was the King of the Ball.

Inside I didn't even take off my coat or my gloves. I'd felt certain haughtiness that one is bound to feel when one has taken in the streets and carpeted pub floors of London as well as this spectacle in the same week. The Rooftops were playing Beatles covers mixed with their own Beatles knock-offs and the guys would push each other onto groups of girls. Courting at its finest. It worked every time. I was amused like a parent is amused, like royalty are amused.

The after party was at Gomba's house, a huge three-storey funkis house with an observatory on top. Gomba was very beautiful, plump with short blond hair in the style of Mia Farrow in *Rosemary's Baby*. All the girls had that hairstyle in Akureyri in '74. I still had my coat on but now at least my gloves were in my pocket. We were talking and smoking. Mostly smoking. I had a burning sensation in my eyes and a shitty taste in my mouth so I tried to drink red wine in big swigs to rinse it out. We talked for a long time and sometimes I would go refill my glass in the kitchen and sometimes she'd have to go to the bathroom or somewhere but we would always come back to the same spot on top of the stairs overlooking the living room.

Her father was a senator and a banker and the house was filled with all sorts of tokens of wealth. Persian rugs and oil paintings. The keen eye could also have detected some indications of the unhealthy relationship between the public and private sectors in our town. Gomba's father was regularly given all sorts of trophies or ornaments from the town's biggest businesses, for his birthday or wedding. Their house had a sauna in the basement, which was quite unheard of. Then there were the souvenirs. Nobody traveled abroad during these years and if you did you went no further than Copenhagen or the harbor cities in Britain and Germany, like Hull, Grimsby, Hamburg, or Cuxhaven. These people had holy water in a bottle from a trip to Jerusalem, and a small roulette trinket from Monaco. Apparently the casinos sent a limo after the old man whenever he was in town on account of his gambling enthusiasm.

Gomba and I were running out of things to say and I kept thinking about the right moment to kiss her. Time wasn't on my side. I was sobering up and pale blue daylight was already streaming through the window. There was a real-life hippie sitting on the sofa with long hair, an open shirt exposing chest hair and lots of jewelry made from wooden beads and turquoise. He was trying to smoke hashish from a pipe while five or six people looked on in amazement. I had never seen anyone smoke hashish before and I had serious doubts regarding whether it had ever reached our town to begin with. There were news stories about the police busting some minor attempt at smuggling or some teenagers carrying small amounts. It was always revealed that the substance was licorice, incense, and dirt. Depressing. But here was the opportunity to make a move on Gomba as the hippie was smoking his hashish and describing the effects to the onlookers with slow wavy hand gestures. We were turned in the same direction and I put my arm around her waist. She looked at me and smiled and then turned her head back towards the living room.

We stood like that for a while. Then she turned around and faced me and put a hand on my shoulder. Our faces were almost together, her eyes turned down towards my lips. Then we heard a chant. First one or two voices and then everyone in the sofa calling loudly towards us "Fuck her! Fuck her! Fuck her!" Even her friends were in on it, making their hands into bugles so they would be louder. Gomba disentangled herself, laughed and made some dismissive gesture. I tried to laugh too. Gomba went down the stairs and joined her friends and everyone, including her, thought this little prank had been absolutely hilarious.

I stayed on for a while but Gomba didn't come back to talk to me. I was developing a headache. I looked at myself in a mirror in a corridor. I looked like shit, with a flushed puffy face and bloodshot eyes. I felt silly in the nice clothes now. I waved goodbye to the small crowd in the living room and hurried out.

A year later I started college in Reykjavík and I heard Gomba had moved to New York. Three years later I met my wife, finished my degree and we moved to Lund in Sweden. I would often think about Gomba in the years after and what could have been. Even that felt like profound betrayal, deeper than fantasizing about another woman, although that was an important component. It was fantasizing about another family, other children and other in-laws, a whole different set of experiences.

I often wondered who had started that chant. It didn't really matter but I always suspected that hippie. It therefore gave me great pleasure some thirty years after the incident when I saw his face on the front of a newspaper. He was the owner and manager of a bed and breakfast in an even smaller town than Akureyri and was arrested for having installed small cameras in the showers and bathrooms of his establishment. Apparently some tourist women noticed a small lens somewhere between the panels in the ceiling. His utter disgrace gave me satisfaction, as well as the fact that the years hadn't treated him very well: he'd turned into a fat bastard.

Shortly after we settled in Lund I was at a café. With an outside terrace. A sign on the door read "Balkongen."

Then it hit me. Balkongen meant balcony, not the King of the Ball.

I thought of Gomba and felt cheated, then guilty, then sad.

The editing of "The King of the Ball"

The following text displays major edits, and other smaller changes can be seen in direct comparison with the published material. Here we can see the work of three editors. The previously mentioned "retrieved" content is indicated with footnote references and in a different font.

In the small town of Akureyri in Iceland, the sixties didn't arrive until we were already almost halfway into the seventies. What's more, not ~~all~~ **much** of the revolutionary spirit of the sixties made it **through?** intact. ~~beyond~~ **Only** some new music and different hairstyles. My generation's parents ~~had~~ belonged to the old system of farmers and fishermen.~~They~~ **who** had been the ones that moved to the town from the surrounding rural areas and still remembered ~~genuine poverty,~~ having to use an outhouse or a bedpan and not having electricity. ~~We remembered those things indirectly from being told about them non-stop~~ **Or so were we told, over and over,** through our childhoods. We were therefore genuinely grateful for all the modern comforts and ~~weren't about to make~~ **wouldn't even think of making** a fuss over things like social stratification or the Viet Nam war. People who are grateful like that tend to be quite conservative.

As the truism would have it, people grew up faster back then. Looking at my old class photo from when we graduated from ~~10th~~ **tenth** grade, everyone seemed really grown up. The men looked like proper adults, most in dark brown or black suits, some with sideburns, some even with full beards, even if ~~most of them~~ **they** were only 16 or 17. The teacher was sitting a little to the left of the group. He had large black-rimmed glasses and looked a lot like Carlos the Jackal. ~~In spite of that he didn't really stand out as the oldest in the bunch.~~

At school, agents, spokespersons or delegates from different organizations or companies had full access to students during school hours. These visits were heartily welcomed by teachers and students alike since the normal curriculum was often repetitive and dull. In the space of a single school year our class would be given over to all sorts delegates and officials on a regular basis.~~: s~~ **S**omeone from the Gideons International would hand out copies of the new testament and say a few words about the benefits of letting Jesus Christ into our lives. A man from the Independence party warned against the devastating effect on our frail economy if taxes or wages would be raised ~~and a man~~[1] **Númi Þorkell** from the YMCA hunted for volunteers both for the nearby lakeside boys' summer camp as well as the mission in Kenya.

The most memorable visit was an emissary from the Good Templars, which was quite a formidable organization in our town. This **small and jittery** man was around 60, ~~small and jittery~~ and had a frown on his face like a mouse looking upwards to sniff at something. He played us a short silent movie using the school's huge projector and every now and then described to us what was happening on the screen in short agitated bursts of speech. The film was Scandinavian, titled "Balkongen," or, as the man translated it, "The King of the Ball." In our dialect, the word "ball" wasn't just used for formal dances but for any type of get-togethers with music and drinks. The film showed a house party in an apartment block with people drinking, playing records and a few dancing in a clunky, awkward way. The film seemed to have a lot of dialogue but our narrator waited patiently through those with his hands crossed over his groin. ~~Once h~~**H**e sprang into motion when a dark haired man entered the frame. "There he is! The King of the Ball!"

He tapped the textile projector screen hard with his finger, denting the picture.

"Look at him!~~" he said almost snarling with indignation, every now and then when that man appeared on the screen.~~ "He's totally deranged from drink. You'll see where that gets you."[2]

The King of the Ball was a normal looking fellow in a light colored suit. He had a drink in his hand and smiled a lot but ~~then again, he seemed to be a minor character in the story. He~~ he didn't participate in any of the dialogues and was mostly seen in the background or in panoramic shots of the party. The short film reached its tragic crescendo during a scene where two women had a heated argument, which lead to one of them falling off the balcony.

~~"Look! This is what you get when you consort with the The King of the Ball!"~~

The old **Templar guy** ~~man~~ tapped on the poor woman who was lying on the pavement below. She raised her head slightly to look up towards the balcony and

---

1   Durneen: "To avoid repetition the man could be named."
2   Durneen: "Without the deleted line, there's more of a contrast between the Templar guy's perspective and the narrator's more balanced 'he was a normal looking fellow.'"

some terrified guests before falling back down lifeless, dramatically succumbing to her injuries. **"This is what you get when you consort with the King of the Ball!"**

But t~~T~~he King of the Ball hadn't been on screen in a while and he wasn't seen again until the guests were all filing out of the building looking somber and miserable. The Templar gave the screen a slightly softer tap this time. "He must be really happy with himself now, the king."

Credits rolled.

After a dramatic pause the old man waxed poetic and asked us to think about the hundreds of seeds that would never become flowers because of The King of the Ball and others of his ilk. **Then he** ~~He then~~ thanked the teacher, said his goodbyes and disappeared with his two huge reels of film in their metal casings. The teetotaler message was mostly lost on us. The film was more confusing than inspiring but I think most of the boys in class that day where left harboring a secret wish to some day become the King of the Ball.

*   *   *

The years after I finished the tenth grade went by quickly. I started going out to sea with my father who was the captain on a fishing trawler. I had been going every now and then during summers since I was ten, more to spend time with my father than to do work, but the crew were quick to find uses for me so I mostly ran around the ship with the ship's dog, Lárpera, and fetched things, sharpened knives, helped mend the nets or delivered messages. Spending time with my father was also nice ~~since me and my siblings had by then begun perceiving him as a distant uncle rather than a close relative~~. He was **almost** always out at sea and when he came home the atmosphere was tense and he mostly wanted to be left alone in his study. The first time he was home at Christmas I was already thirteen and it felt strange to see someone else sitting in my mother's chair.

After the tenth grade I was out at sea so much ~~that missing out became the norm, especially around summers and holidays. Over the space of several years~~ I missed out on countless parties, camping trips and friends' weddings. I also both missed out on the not-yet-so-famous Kinks playing in our local movie theater and later I also missed out on Led Zeppelin, playing a packed show in our giant handball arena at the peak of their career. It was perhaps no big surprise then that the King of the Ball loomed large in my thoughts during this time.

A chance presented itself when the crew found itself in the small harbor city of Hull with a few days' shore leave. The plan was to leave the old trawler to be scrapped and then sail home on a brand new one. My father was busy with moving equipment between the two trawlers and the rest of the crew would ~~go sleep with~~ **visit** prostitutes and get anchors tattooed on their forearms marking the occasion, with "Hull 1974" inscribed beneath. The first thing I did was to get on the next train to London. At Piccadilly Circus I walked straight into Aquascutum, which sold high quality clothes for gentlemen, and proceeded to dress myself up like the king. I bought a suit and an overcoat and some dress shirts, shoes, leather gloves, a belt, and a scarf. It cost around two months' wages but I didn't care. I was always working and I never had a chance to spend anything. ~~so it didn't matter. I then spent the next two days going to pubs and museums and walking around the city, before returning to Hull and our new trawler.~~ A week later we were docking again back home. Akureyri had never seemed smaller and the mountains around it had never seemed bigger and more imposing. Seeing the dockworkers and the old cars parked nearby made me feel like I had just traveled back in time.

~~I didn't get in touch with anyone of my friends. Most of them were renting rooms somewhere and had access to telephones but it was a Friday night most likely everyone was out somewhere.~~ As I walked back home over the gravel lot with the taxis I could see posters advertising a ball that very evening, with a band playing and everything. This was my chance. I got dressed in my new clothes and drove to the ball. I sat in my car for a while close to the venue, our handball arena, and listened to the national radio. ~~A program was on called~~ Sailors' Requests **was on,** mostly play**ing** upbeat accordion music. I took swigs from a small vodka bottle and smoked Royale cigarettes. I had grown quite tall and the roof of my Volkswagen beetle flattened the top of my Afro hairdo. When I had polished off the vodka I got out and walked towards the arena.

It was the time of year, which our poet had described as the time between hay and grass. ~~Historically this was the time of year when men and animals would drop like flies since the previous summer's hay had finished but the spring grass hadn't started showing.~~

It was the time of year, which our poet, Halldór Laxness, had described as the time between hay and grass, when winter was supposed to be over but spring was not in sight, and men and animals used to drop like flies. This was in the olden days, which in Iceland lasted until WWII, when the blessed war made everyone rich and modern.[3]

The air was cold and crisp and after six weeks of diesel fumes I felt I could smell the oxygen in the air. The cold didn't come with the wind but rather seemed to radiate from the ground and the yellow grass was frozen so it made a soft creaking sound when you walked on it.

There was already a line outside the venue. Most of the people were dressed up but a few of the men seemed to have just headed there straight after work. They looked like the dockworkers ~~I had~~ **I'd** seen earlier~~;~~ **–** in dirty and worn woolen sweaters with sixpence caps and specks of course snuff tobacco around their noses and mouths~~. Seeing this group I could~~ **– and they made me** feel the sort of confidence that's born out of sheer contempt for one's fellow man. I was also drunk and looking like a goddamned prince. I walked past the line and went straight inside. I didn't even stop to pay for a ticket. ~~I had momentum;~~ I was the King of the Ball.

---

3   Durneen suggested the above cut because the text was not clear, but after a discussion we came to realise the information was needed, only the paragraph needed to be reworked as shown.

Inside **I didn't even take off my coat or my gloves. I had felt a certain haughtiness that one is bound to feel when one has taken in the streets and carpeted pub floors of London as well as this spectacle in the same week.** ~~the evening turned into a haze. I met some of my friends. There was hugging and bits of conversation screamed into each other's ear.~~ The Rooftops were playing Beatles covers mixed with their own Beatles knock-offs and ~~. The men would approach women in total cave man fashion. The most time-tried tactic was to have a friend push you onto a group of girls. When you crashed into them you had to be super sensitive to the groups reaction because chances were one of the girls wouldn't push back quite as hard as the others. I didn't participate in any of this.~~ **the guys would push each other onto groups of girls. It worked every time.**[4] I was amused like a parent is amused, like royalty is amused.

~~I didn't really snap out of it until I had been at the after party for a while.~~ The after party was at Gomba's house, a huge three-storey funkis house with an observatory on top. Gomba ~~and I were talking. She~~ was very beautiful, plump with short blond hair in the style of Mia Farrow in *Rosemary's Baby*. All the girls had that hairstyle in Akureyri in '74. I still had my coat on but now at least my gloves were in the pocket. We were talking and smoking. Mostly smoking. I had a burning sensation in my eyes and a shitty taste in my mouth so I tried to drink red wine in big swigs to rinse it out. We talked for a long time and sometimes I would go refill my glass in the kitchen and sometimes she'd have to go to the bathroom or somewhere but we would always come back to ~~this~~ **the same** spot on top of the stairs overlooking the living room.

Her father was a senator and a banker and the house was filled with all sorts of tokens of wealth. ~~, such as statues,~~ Persian rugs and oil paintings. The keen eye could also have detected some tokens of the unhealthy relationship between the public and private sectors in our town. ~~Gomba's father was regularly given all sorts of trophies or ornaments from the town's biggest businesses, for his birthday or wedding anniversary: a carved walrus tooth on a cubic marble foundation with a silver placard, or a detailed porcelain falcon with a congratulatory greeting engraved on its base.~~ Their house had a sauna in the basement, which was quite unheard of**. Then there** ~~but the biggest symbol of their wealth~~ were the souvenirs. Nobody traveled abroad during these years and if you did you went no further than Copenhagen or the harbor cities in Britain and Germany, like Hull, Grimsby, Hamburg, or Cuxhaven. These people had holy water in a bottle from a trip to Jerusalem, and a small roulette trinket from Monaco. Apparently the casinos sent a limo after the old man whenever he was in town on account of his gambling enthusiasm.

Gomba and I were running out of things to say and I kept thinking about the right moment to give her a kiss. Time wasn't on my side. I was sobering up and pale blue daylight was already streaming through the window. ~~We stood in silence and looked at the crowd in the party.~~ There was a real-life ~~genuine~~ hippie sitting on the

---

4   The same issue was the case in this cut. We wanted to bring back the scene but it had
    to be rewritten as shown to avoid overwriting.

sofa with long hair, an open shirt exposing chest hair and lots of jewelry made from wooden beads and turquoise. He was trying to smoke hashish from a pipe ~~and~~ while five or six people looked on in amazement. I had never seen anyone smoke hashish before and I had serious doubts regarding whether it had ever reached our town to begin with. ~~There were news stories every now and then about the police busting some minor attempt at smuggling or some teenagers carrying small amounts. It was always revealed in the end that the substance in question was either licorice, incense, dirt or any combination of the three. For some reason I often found those news depressing. T~~ **There were news stories about the police busting some minor attempt at smuggling or some teenagers carrying small amounts. It was always revealed that the substance was licorice, incense, and dirt. Depressing.**[5] **But here was t**he opportunity to make a move on Gomba, ~~arose~~ as the hippie was smoking his hashish and describing the effects to the onlookers with slow wavy hand gestures. We were turned in the same direction and I put my arm around her waist. She looked at me and smiled and then turned her head back towards the living room. We stood like that for a while. ~~When nothing interesting seemed to be going on Gomba~~ **Then she** turned around and faced me and put a hand on my shoulder. ~~She hugged me and withdrew so~~ our **Our** faces were almost together, her eyes turned down towards my lips. Then we heard a chant. First one or two voices and then everyone in the sofa calling loudly towards us "Fuck her! Fuck her! Fuck her!" Even her friends were in on it, making their hands into bugles so they would be louder. Gomba disentangled herself, ~~looked down at the people,~~ laughed and made some dismissive gesture. I tried to laugh too. Gomba went down the stairs and joined her friends and everyone, including her, thought this little prank had been absolutely hilarious.

I stayed on for a while but Gomba didn't **come back** to talk to me. I was developing a headache. I took a look at myself in a mirror in a corridor. I looked like shit, with a flushed puffy face and bloodshot eyes. I felt very silly in the nice clothes now. I waved goodbye to the small crowd in the living room as I hurried out.

* * *

~~Aside from a couple of awkward encounters, Gomba and I didn't really cross paths after that evening and a a~~ **A** year later I had started college in a slightly bigger city in the North and **I heard Gomba** ~~she~~ had moved to New York. Three years later I met my wife, finished my degree and we moved to Lund in Sweden based on the logic that it was so close to Copenhagen (strangely enough, we didn't just move to Copenhagen where we could be close to Lund).[6] **A year later I started college**

---

5 In this case, as before, the information Durneen cut was brought back into the text with slight changes.
6 Durneen wrote: "Not sure this is needed? What's important about either Copenhagen or Lund?" The passage was then rewritten as shown.

in Reykjavík and I heard Gomba had moved to New York. Three years later I met my wife, finished my degree and we moved to Lund in Sweden. I would often think about Gomba in the years after and what could have been. ~~Just thinking about~~ **Even that** felt like profound betrayal, ~~. The betrayal went~~ deeper than fantasizing about another woman, although that was an important component. It was fantasizing about another family, other children and other in-laws, a whole different set of experiences. ~~Whenever I saw anything that stood out as luxurious or exotic my mind would go back to Gomba and I would feel cheated, then sad, then guilty.~~

I often ~~thought of~~ **wondered** who had started that chant. It didn't really matter but I had always suspected that hippie. It therefore gave me great pleasure some thirty years after the incident when I saw his face on front of a newspaper. He had been the owner and operator of a bed and breakfast in an even smaller town than Akureyri and had been arrested for having installed small cameras in the showers and bathrooms of his establishment. Apparently some tourist women had noticed a small lens somewhere between the panels in the ceiling. His utter disgrace gave me pleasure, as well as the fact that the years hadn't treated him very well: he had turned into a fat bastard.

~~The most important piece of the whole puzzle fell into place s~~**S**hortly after we settled in Lund I was at a café ~~that had a door leading to~~ **with** an outside terrace. A sign on the door read "Balkongen." Then it hit me. Balkongen meant "balcony", not 'the king of the ball'.

I thought of Gomba and I felt cheated, then guilty, then sad.

~~I hadn't thought about that film and that old man from the Good Templars in years. I was stunned. Why would anyone go around playing a short film about a balcony to teenagers and make up this extraordinary figure, this King of the Ball? I seriously entertained the idea that the old mouse-faced guy had been Satan himself. He was the one that planted this extraordinary idea in my head, tempted me, helped prop me up as this mock king who was then set up for failure and humiliated.~~

~~The more I thought about it the more my anger and confusion subsided and a new feeling took over. It was pity, sympathy and warmth, all at once, for this poor old man who had stumbled upon an artsy short film and misunderstood it so absolutely and with so much fervor. It felt good to live in a world were a mouse-faced man could roam the countryside and ripple the water a little in the minds of the young.~~

Conversation about "The King of the Ball"
Friðrik Sólnes Jónsson, Lucy Durneen and Adnan Mahmutović

I think it is important to preface this case with some history of our professional relationship, which Lucy and I could see was very important in other cases in this book. Since 2012, I have taught Friðrik in literary studies, culture studies, and creative writing. We recently co-published an article on Roberto Bolano. When it comes to writer-editor type of engagement, I have worked with Friðrik on his first published story "Ferðasaga" (*Two Thirds North* 2013), so when he submitted "The King of the Ball" in 2015, I was quite familiar with his themes and writing style. I have always been impressed by his sense of humor, but sometimes found the prose to be over-written. However, at *Two Thirds North*, we are keen on fresh, authentic stories, even if they require substantial editorial work. Our previous work on "Ferðasaga" mainly involved cutting, some minor restructuring, and tightening the ending.

Durneen

I want to also pick up on the question of that relationship. As you say, it is becoming increasingly clear that it is a very unique thing, an essential part of the process of negotiation in our other cases, and I'm wondering if that makes one more, or less, prepared to trust in the editorial suggestions.

Sólnes Jónsson

First off, there was an interesting difference in my whole attitude towards editing during our work on "Ferðasaga" and "The King of the Ball." With "Ferðasaga," I was taken aback by the extent of changes Adnan suggested. I thought I had been very thorough myself. I had spent a lot of time editing and revising with help from my smart friend Viðar. We had been exchanging drafts and discussing it over Skype. I was very surprised when Adnan suggested huge cuts, and worse to my mind, offered an entirely new ending. There were also suggestions for new lines of dialogue. In Iceland I have personally enjoyed considerable freedom, and often completely free rein, with my own projects, such as my prologues, reviews, and articles. Also, in this specific case, I was a bit shocked to see at least three editors tampering with my story – not only editing, as in "cutting fat," but using it as a platform to try out ideas of their own by writing bits of dialogue or alternative endings.

At the time we worked on "The King of the Ball," I was a lot more attuned to the fact that this was a process and the story would undergo a lot of change, especially since I was a bit pressed for time and submitted something that I felt was hastily put together. In other words, I personally did far less editing on this story, but I suppose a few years of experience between my first and this story does make a difference. Besides, between working on these two stories I have taken some of Adnan's creative writing courses as well as his Editing & Publishing MA module where I even got to experience the frustration of having to argue my own edits with a writer whose work we accepted for publication.

Durneen

So, thinking of "Ferðasaga" just for a minute, you had the experience of a significantly more interventionist approach. Not only cuts, but additions, a kind of grafting of another writer's suggestions on to your own piece. There's another thing too, which is the move between literary languages. We're moving from one of the smallest – Icelandic – to one of the largest – English – and you're working in your second language here too. I am just thinking that this must make it quite difficult to know what instincts to trust. The question is, how to preserve your own aesthetic whilst also evaluating the benefits of the proposed changes?

Sólnes Jónsson

As for my own experience, I wrote a prologue once for my comic writer friend. A proofreader changed a word, or rather the gender of a word (I was talking about *drakmas* and *kopeks*) and this annoyed me so I asked that the next prologue not be proofread at all. That was granted without a peep like I was Barbara Cartland or somebody. But then again, with "The King of the Ball," I came to the table thinking beforehand that I was going to accept most or all of the suggestions. I did argue against some changes though, but my daughter Malla had been screaming at me and I did not have any fight left in me to hold out.

I think our work on "Ferðasaga" had more to do with the move from Icelandic to English than "King of the Ball." "Ferðasaga" was my first attempt at creative writing in English and a project that used notes and (mostly fictional) diaries I had written in Icelandic. The transition into English revealed several problem areas, such as an excessive use of the pluperfect verb form, which would be more acceptable in Icelandic, and an odd choice of words here and there. When I write in Icelandic I like to play around with voice, imagery and sometimes use archaisms but when I translate this style of writing wholesale into English, the effects can sometimes be off-putting. This wasn't as much of an issue with "The King of the Ball" because I wrote it all in English and made a very conscious decision that the Icelandic exoticism would be restricted to the level of content, such as the elements we mentioned above regarding the specificity of the setting – the hashish, the courting etc. This is also why I thought it was important that these details were kept in the story.

Mahmutović

Yes, I do not recall much argument. You pretty much wrote that you trust the English lady. Her word is my law. (I just want to add that having had a longish history with you I wanted the input of an outsider I trusted. A fresh pair of eyes.)

Sólnes Jónsson

Yes, I did not argue a lot there. And that was totally the right decision.

Mahmutović

You seemed more afraid of her image, which I may or may not have created.

Sólnes Jónsson

Yes there was that too.

Mahmutović

Initially you had particular issues with Lucy's edit? What sorts of things did you feel were spot on and what were you unsure about?

Sólnes Jónsson

I remember the only significant edits I was not sure about were the culturally specific details. Lucy wanted to cut many of those but I thought the details were important.

Durneen

Something I am interested in here, and which we might come back to at some point, is that element of trust. For example, it might be a sweeping question but does writing in a second language make a writer more susceptible to just assuming the editor, like Adnan or myself, is always right?

But is (absolute) trust in an editor a good thing? Should there be a healthy resistance to suggestions, which, as Adnan and I have seen in throughout all the different cases, are often reconsidered and retracted by both editor and writer? And this then leads into that other, hard to qualify territory – what Adnan has called our different instincts about essential vs. inessential content. This too has come up in other cases. What is essential? To whom?

Thinking of "The King of the Ball," my first reading of it was that this was a story that *had* to be taken, though that decision was already made by Adnan's team. And yet, I felt that it *did* need editing, in a way that some stories do not (that is not a reflection on quality, but a sense that you almost did not see quite how good a story it was. It just needed a little helping out of the chrysalis, so to speak).

So for me, essentiality became about revealing the real story, which I felt was sometimes obscured by details. They were authentic details, sure. Perhaps as Adnan says with "Ferðasaga," they just got in the way of storytelling.

Here's an example from page two:

> He tapped the textile projector screen hard with his finger, denting the picture. "Look at him! ~~he said almost snarling with indignation, every now and then when that man appeared on the screen~~. He's totally deranged from drink. You'll see where that gets you." The King of the Ball was a normal looking fellow in a light colored suit . . .

My original comment was: Without the deleted line, there is more of a contrast between the Templar guy's perspective and the narrator's more balanced "he was a normal looking fellow."

You see, for me, this was not just inessential information, but the extra detail actually obscured the contrast. Then a few lines down we took out this line: "This is what you get when you consort with the King of the Ball!"

Sólnes Jónsson

Also, that "snarling with indignation" reads a bit like overwriting. Like "he refuted fervently" type of thing.

Durneen

Same reason. And actually, this is about another issue of trust: trust between writer and reader. The fact that you do not need to necessarily explain how to interpret things. We could put "snarling" on our proscribed, over-used words list along with "shards" and "pearlescent."

Sólnes Jónsson

Probably "indignation" too.

Durneen

Quite. Ok, so let us look at this example. The original read as follows:

> It was the time of year, which our poet had described as the time between hay and grass. ~~Historically this was the time of year when men and animals would drop like flies since the previous summer's hay had finished but the spring grass hadn't started showing.~~

I cut the second sentence, and then, after your deliberation, it became:

> It was the time of year, which our poet, Halldór Laxness, had described as the time between hay and grass, when winter was supposed to be over but spring was not in sight, and men and animals used to drop like flies. This was in the olden days, which in Iceland lasted until WWII, when the blessed war made everyone rich and modern.

This example is interesting because we can see how you responded and how it might reflect the interpretation of essential and inessential. I took out the explanation of what the "time between hay and grass" means, mainly because it is clear that it is a cultural reference (although I am not familiar with the expression), and the meaning is implicit enough that it does not confuse me. I deemed that inessential, and perhaps just a little too expositional. Specifically, it is the "Historically this was the time of year" that creates that effect.

You effectively put it all back in, and are right to do so, but it is changed. It becomes more concrete in that "our poet" becomes "our poet, Halldór Laxness," and the listing of what happens at this time of year feels more lyrical, less telegraphed. The new line "This was in the olden days, which in Iceland lasted until WWII, when the blessed war made everyone rich and modern" gives context without announcing it is going to give context.

Sólnes Jónsson

So you agree with the final inclusion of it? By assigning it to Laxness?

Durneen

Absolutely.

Mahmutović

Exactly, when we discussed this and decided to bring it back into the text I asked Friðrik to rewrite it and then I edited it some more (as I did with much of the resurrected text). I understood why Lucy cut it in the first place, but I also realized that it was not just about inessential info but the way it was presented. Not the content but the form, the delivery.

Durneen

It turns out that it was not the detail that was inessential, but rather that the framing of it was getting in the way of the storytelling. In fact, the new version *makes* it essential. It is really important that this event happens at a threshold time for the narrator, both in terms of the world around him and his own, more particular, experience.

Mahmutović

Here we have an example of a risk we are running as editors. We see that something does not work, and we judge that something is inessential while it is merely unsuccessfully executed.

My first instinct was not different from yours, Lucy, so it to took some rewriting to get it right. I think this editorial error, if we want to call it that, has to do with the default notion we share that editing is essentially cutting, or pruning, and seldom addition, rewriting, etc. As we write in our introduction, the reality is most often that we do not really have the time to get personally involved in deeper rewrites. I feel I do that many times if I do not have the kind of working relationship with an author like I do with you two. Even though at *Two Thirds North* we have often accepted stories that were diamonds in the rough, truth is one cannot afford the time required for that "let it breathe" comment Robert Gottlieb would offer.

Durneen

Not only do we not have time for deep rewrites, that becomes something else. It risks being intrusive. It risks what we might call 'doing a Gordon Lish'.

Mahmutović

Not necessarily Lish, but yes, there is a risk. In the case of "Ferðasaga," that story came through my workshop so I was already very familiar with the text and felt I could be more intrusive, as you say, because it was between that and rejecting the story. I expected to have to talk things through and in fact the ending I suggested was just a way, as I wrote in my comment to Friðrik, of exemplifying what needed to be done. The ending he then wrote contains bits of that ending and a great deal more which closed the story the way it needed to be closed.

When I received "The King of the Ball," my instinct was not to do the same thing I did before, which I suspected I would do. So I decided to give it to you, Lucy. For you, it would be like any other story you would get through submissions, anonymous really. I did not even mention I knew the author and why I wanted you to edit it.

Durneen

Yes, I wonder how I would have approached the editing of it now. We saw this with Passaro and Drew. They have a kind of shorthand that is clearly evolved between them.

When an editor understands the aesthetic of the writer they are working with, it is easier to nudge them towards what really needs to be said, but sometime you could be too close as well.

Mahmutović

I think working off your initial instinct was good. It turned out well, exactly because you highlighted the seemingly inessential passages and I knew that if we wanted to fight for those we needed to find a solution rather than just reject your cuts. In other words, it was not wrong what you did, but it shows the complexity of the process, something which does not always get practiced. So, the moral is, both trust and distrust the English lady.

Durneen

As I think has been the lesson we might learn from history regarding the English.

Mahmutović

What is important is that which you mentioned earlier: the fact that Friðrik did not really see how good the story was. Anna Crofts, our assistant editor, you, and I, recognized this while Friðrik kept thinking it was very rough. But at the same time he was right, it needed editing. It was rough around the edges and that pushed you to those kinds of edits.

Durneen

Yes. From an editing POV, it was actually more rewarding. Super-polished pieces save time, but perhaps could themselves still be even better – it is just harder to see where you need to push them.

Mahmutović

What we can learn from Robin Hemley's case is how his editor Jennifer Sahn was not quick to cut everything that felt inessential to her, but asked him to reconsider or rewrite or argue for keeping something.

Durneen

Yes, the quiz especially. When it came down to it, he could not argue a strong enough case for it, and its inessentiality became obvious.

Mahmutović

She let it breathe, in a way. I have to say, when I edit your stories, Lucy, I feel I have a better grasp of the inessential because I know that if it is just the form, the language, etc., you can fix it.

 Now, let us look at other examples where material was brought back into the text.

Sólnes Jónsson

There are mainly three details that Lucy cut and we went on to discuss: the hashish, Gomba's father's ornaments and then the crashing into girls bit.

Durneen

For me, the crashing into girls bit was too dense. Too distracting. They are pushing into a group of girls? And then the girls do what? It prompted me to start trying to unravel the exact choreography of this when really the only important thing was: the boys had a really basic way of hitting on the girls, but it worked.

Sólnes Jónsson

Here is that larger section where the part in bold letters is the reinsertion of the (somewhat rewritten) material:

> Gomba and I were running out of things to say and I kept thinking about the right moment to give her a kiss. Time wasn't on my side. I was sobering up and pale blue daylight was already streaming through the window. ~~We stood in silence and looked at the crowd in the party.~~ There was a real-life ~~genuine~~ hippie sitting on the sofa with long hair, an open shirt exposing chest hair and lots of jewelry made from wooden beads and turquoise. He was trying to smoke hashish from a pipe ~~and~~ while five or six people looked on in amazement. I had never seen anyone smoke hashish before and I had serious doubts regarding whether it had ever reached our town to begin with. ~~There were news stories every now and then about the police busting some minor attempt at smuggling or some teenagers carrying small amounts. It was always revealed in the end that the substance in question was either licorice, incense, dirt or any combination of the three. For some reason I often found those news depressing. T~~ **There were news stories about the police busting some minor attempt at smuggling or some teenagers carrying small amounts. It was always revealed that the substance was licorice, incense, and dirt. Depressing. But here was t**he opportunity to make a move on Gomba, ~~arose~~ as the hippie was smoking his hashish and describing the effects to the onlookers with slow, wavy hand gestures.

That standalone "depressing" is the one thing in the final version I'm still unhappy about.

Mahmutović

I like it. It is good for the sake of change in the rhythm, a necessary pause, and, it has a bit of a comedic effect, which I thought was suitable. Like exaggerated emphasis.

Durneen

I think what these cuts have in common (Gomba's father too) is that they kind of offroad the real story.

Mahmutović

Now I wonder, Lucy, in this part you questioned the importance of Copenhagen and Lund:

> A year later I had started college in a slightly bigger city in the North and I heard Gomba she had moved to New York. Three years later I met my wife,

finished my degree and we moved to Lund in Sweden based on the logic that it was so close to Copenhagen (strangely enough, we didn't just move to Copenhagen where we could be close to Lund).

It was then rewritten:

A year later I started college in Reykjavík and I heard Gomba had moved to New York. Three years later I met my wife, finished my degree and we moved to Lund in Sweden.

Durneen

It is about pinning down what is relevant to the story. With the boys pushing girls it is the basic crudeness of their flirting techniques. With the hashish it is that it is often not really hashish. With Copenhagen/Lund it is that one day the narrator moves to Sweden and it is there that he understands the real meaning of Balkongen. It is about the fact he has a new life, not the minutiae of it. It could be Stockholm, it could be Tranås, it does not matter. What matters is the epiphany.

Sólnes Jónsson

I think the root of the issue might be what you mentioned earlier. I maybe did not have a lot of faith in the story itself so I thought it would need to rely more on the setting, the exotic allure of a backwards small town. The Copenhagen/Lund thing has to do with the fact that for 95% of Icelanders going abroad meant going to one of those two places to study.

Durneen

But that's where, in a way, you are getting distracted by making it real, instead of an approximation of reality.

Sólnes Jónsson

I just think it is so depressing, and I thought it emphasized how far away and unattainable Gomba's whole life was to the guy.

Mahmutović

I think it is exactly that specific detail you now mention, that Copenhagen was like Mars for those guys, that is interesting. Otherwise you got no characterization.

Durneen

I'm thinking that too. You know that expression about drama, that the problem with the last act is usually a problem with the first act? If you had mentioned

Copenhagen/Lund as a kind of inevitable destination in the first third, say, it would have a different resonance by the end. Or not inevitable, I mean, like Mars. So again – not inessential, as it turns out, just about presentation and form.

Sólnes Jónsson

I think the thought experiment, or even real exercise of stripping down specificity helps you see what is essential.

Durneen

Yes.

Sólnes Jónsson

But maybe it has to do with essential stuff and cultural opacity by degrees. I am sure some of my fellow countrymen, especially those of my parents' generation would read differently into place names like Lund. So perhaps it needed more presence in the story, not less. This is a huge debate in world lit. Whether more modernist abstract writing means better ability to travel and more realist writing means less travelling.

Durneen

Specificity all the way.

Mahmutović

Well you had editors from at least three nations and abstract was not what appealed to us.

I represent two nations, by the way, but Anna Crofts was in on it as well, so Sweden was twice represented.

Durneen

We need to talk about the ending particularly. I cut this entire section:

> I hadn't thought about that film and that old man from the Good Templars in years. I was stunned. Why would anyone go around playing a short film about a balcony to teenagers and make up this extraordinary figure, this King of the Ball? I seriously entertained the idea that the old mouse-faced guy had been Satan himself. He was the one that planted this extraordinary idea in my head, tempted me, helped prop me up as this mock king who was then set up for failure and humiliated.

~~The more I thought about it the more my anger and confusion subsided and a new feeling took over. It was pity, sympathy and warmth, all at once, for this poor old man who had stumbled upon an artsy short film and misunderstood it so absolutely and with so much fervor. It felt good to live in a world were a mouse-faced man could roam the countryside and ripple the water a little in the minds of the young.~~

Sólnes Jónsson

Yes, the ending was the arguably the worst written part of the first manuscript.

Durneen

Being technical about it, I felt it corresponded to Susan Lohafer's ideas of *preclosure*. Lohafer says of *preclosure* that there's a point in the story which the reader thinks is the end. She explored what readers felt when the story extended beyond that point.

The story had already ended with the *balcony* epiphany. These last paragraphs were more consciously reflexive. They were doing the work of the reader. And for me, the saddest thing about the story, the part that really moved me, was the narrator's non-relationship with Gomba and how the memory of it was stronger and more impacting than the reality of what it had been. So I felt it needed to end with her.

There's that saying about how Chekhov says we should cut our first and last paragraphs because "that's where we do most of our lying." For me, the momentum changed. It peaked, with Gomba and the realization of the meaning of balkongen, and then it was like it was trying to get started again, go uphill, and there was no space left in the story to do this.

Mahmutović

OK, let us end on the ending. Thank you all for the conversation.

6

"EVERYTHING I KNOW ABOUT COMIC BOOKS* (*AND WHAT I AM AFRAID TO ASK.)"

World Literature Today, Spring 2015

Lucy Durneen and Adnan Mahmutović

The essence of the editorial process in this case lies in the attempt to help an author to assert her voice and authority over the story as such. By story, we do not mean the final published draft, the text itself, which is always shaped under some authority of the editor. Rather, story here means that which the author is trying to convey. There is a whole set of issues one could highlight in the process of writing-editing Durneen's piece, but what needs to be emphasized above all is the building of trust in the fact that both parties' involvement is essential for the sake of the story and for the sake of creating firmer fundaments for the author to gain authority over her narrative. In other words, the balance does not mean both the author and the editor are equal. The author lies both at the centre and periphery. The editor, even if s/he is a friend, is a tool. The more involved and intimate the relationship may be, the more of a tool the editor becomes. In the following texts, pre-writing chats, and post-publication critical conversation, one can see several examples of the technique of "let it breathe." This advice is, here, more of a metonym for certain types of editorial advice which arise from the fact that the author and the editor understand each other, or rather understand the core of the story that needs to be told. So for instance, when Durneen creates her story around the narrative she heard from her friend, this may indeed be central to what she is trying to convey, but at the same time, the editor needs to see that there is another story unfolding beneath that surface reaction, the story that is the very reason for the precise emotional response to her friend's story. The editor needs to see and convey in the right way that this hidden story is in fact the one that presents the true, the good, and the beautiful of any storytelling. Once that is recognized and affirmed, the rest of the rather typical editing process follows effortlessly. This case teaches us that the mechanics and craft of editing might well arise from that fundamental connection which is neither about craft nor mechanics.

"Everything I know about comic books*
(*and what I am afraid to ask.)"

You're in Forbidden Planet on Burleigh Street, Cambridge, the new, improved store, the world's number one for your comic book needs. This is good, because you've got a comic book need. Up until last year Forbidden Planet was a hushed place on the other side of the street; crossing the threshold was more an admission of something than an intent to purchase. But this new store is a clean well-lighted place and inside, flicking through the browsers of graphic novels, you want to belong. You gaze at the high shelves, the acreage of stories. Some titles are familiar, most not. By familiar you mean the ones with characters your kids wear on their pyjamas.

Your plan is to look like you know what you're doing, because that's what Indiana Jones would do. So when you approach the desk to ask for help in tracking down early 90s Bonelli, but not the Italian ones, the ones from the former Yugoslavia, you assume the casual, professional air of a true collector. This is the way you always spend your lunch breaks. *No time for love, Doctor Jones.*

The assistants at the counter look at you and their beards twitch. What's wrong with Marvel? they want to know. But the word you have fixed on is Bonelli, so you shake your head as if you're disappointed by their lack of knowledge. It has to be early 90s, you say. Really, it has to be from 1992. It has to be from – you find your-self getting tangled up in the geography. The Balkans, you say in the end. You might as well have said Mars. They turn back to setting up a little diorama of Minecraft merchandise. They don't even bother to shake their heads. Try the internet, one of them says.

The internet – where everything and nothing is possible. Like you hadn't already thought of that.

In the summer of 1992 an almost-fifteen-year-old girl and her best friend went to the annual Strawberry Fair in Cambridge, England. The girl thought maybe they would ride the waltzer and pretend to drink lemon Hooch with the kids she hoped might stop giving her a hard time if she acted a little more like them. Instead, outside a dirty canvas tent, she found a bucket of goldfish waiting to be transferred to the cellophane globes on the nearby Hook a Duck stand. The fish looked sad, a seething mass of orange like a solar explosion in a plastic tub. The girl and her friend looked around, picked up the unattended bucket and walked fast until they were two streets away from the fair, water surging over the bucket's lip at every step and soaking the toes of their Doc Marten 8-holes.

The girl was kind of lonely. She read a lot. Too much. The other girls in her class were pretty and were learning how to kiss the boys in the dark of the school drama theatre. The boys in her class made vomiting sounds when they played spin the bottle and the bottle stopped on her. Somewhere around the beginning of 1992 she had decided to stop eating, as if loneliness and food were connected somehow and she could fix one by rationing the other.

The girl watched Tintin on Sunday mornings and scared herself with Twilight Zone and that was as much as she knew about comic books. By the summer of 1992 she hadn't eaten anything except cabbage cooked in vegetable stock for nearly four months. She had a crush on Cyrano de Bergerac. Partly this was because of Gerard Depardieu, who hadn't yet gotten fat and started pissing in planes, but partly because she still half-believed in the existence of heroes that didn't look like heroes, the ones that maybe were OK about it if you got good grades and wrote poems and didn't have big boobs or straight teeth.

One time the girl's mother threw a plate of food at her and shouted, Why can't you just be normal? And she really wanted to know. The girl's father was in the business of reconnaissance. She hadn't seen him for some months. In summer 1992 she didn't actually know where he was, other than that a war in a place that was no longer Yugoslavia had taken him away.

Eventually, officially, wars come to an end. Some people get to go back home, like the girl's father. Mostly war follows you, invisibly, internally. You can make it your business to study the writing of war, but there is always the knowledge, a deep guilt in the regolith of you, that no matter how much you read you can never, actually, know. Lives converge until the moment they absolutely don't.

In the summer of 1992, or thereabouts, another thing was happening, something the girl only hears about more than two decades later, via Facebook messenger. A boy and his best friend pushed a wheelbarrow full of comic books into the mountains above the Bosnian city of Banja Luka to try and hide them from soldiers. Afraid that wild animals would destroy them, they came up with a different plan. Wrapping the comics in plastic bags, they lowered them to safety in a septic tank, only to realise some time later that the bags might not be shitproof. It turned out this was indeed the case. The comics were retrieved. The boy used up a whole can of his mother's expensive deodorant to take away the smell. His mother wanted to kill him. His words.

Twenty-two years later, the boy, now the girl's friend, writes to her and says, I was really stupid, wasn't I?

The girl, you, says, No, and it's not entirely a lie. It's what Indiana Jones would do.

That's how little I was worried about being killed, he says. Bloody geek.

But geeks are so much cooler than nerds.

What?

Sorry. I thought that was my inside voice.

Your eldest son is a proud Doctor Who geek, and inordinately fond of that viral song Dumb Ways to Die. He worries a lot about being killed. By solar flare, freak asteroid impact, zombie apocalypse, Ebola. You try to imagine him navigating checkpoints, hiding his stuff from soldiers, and remember how last time he made lunch for himself he used a tea strainer to drain a can of tuna fish.

When your friend tells you about the comic books in the septic tank, it's like you are watching the scene in a snow globe, or Asimov's chronoscope, these two kids and their wheelbarrow going up one street and down another, their frustration growing, and perhaps also their fear, but he doesn't mention that.

Somewhere in this is the need to change something. If you could shout down through the time vortex. If he could look up into the ether to see you waving. What would you say? Throw me your comics, I'll keep them safe for you? Or – hang on, I'm coming down, let me help push the damn wheelbarrow? A nerdy girl, you think, might have come up with a better plan than a septic tank.

Your friend sends you an essay to read, something he wrote after you met in Vienna last summer. It's about faith and forgiveness. Here you see he's ambivalent about forgiving a person who once stole his collection of Bonelli comics. He's joking, sure, but – there are those comic books again, you think. They really do mean something.

You read the essay about ten times. You want to ask so many things. Bonelli, it says. *Bonelli*. You commit it to memory, which is a less abstruse way of saying it starts to haunt you. Italian. Were these the comics sunk into the septic tank and ravaged by shit and expensive deodorant? You think of that story about Hadley Hemingway, the famous one in which she catches a train to visit Ernest in Lausanne and whilst waiting at the Gare de Lyon her suitcase containing every last one of the original Nick Adams stories is stolen. You imagine the despair of knowing that there is nothing to replace the thing you have lost, an emptiness that stretches out about as long as the journey to Switzerland.

When the idea comes to you, it comes the way anything obvious and also impossible arrives in your mind. You want to replace those ruined comics. You know nothing about Bonelli, but by some chance, you work alongside magical agents and allies. You leave behind the sleek, contemporary corridors of the university in which you teach and cross over to the Victorian halls of the Cambridge School of Art. There are geeks, collectors, and experts on graphic literature in every room, but this one seems out of even their league. Someone knows someone somewhere in Slovenia who maybe once had a thing about comic books. Will that help?

It doesn't. That's how you end up in Forbidden Planet talking to assistants with twitchy beards who'd rather sell you the latest Spider-Man.

When you said you know nothing about comic books this is not entirely true. It's just that you're not talking your Silver Surfer or Blueberry. You're definitely not talking Corto Maltese.

There was a time when you and your friend Sarah were avid devotees of the *Just Seventeen* photo story, which is to say that you were romantics who had not yet experienced romance and were educating yourself on mildly erotic, post-punk tales of attraction featuring bad boys in leather jackets, which explains a lot about your respective emotional crises to come. On one occasion, planning a surreptitious photo shoot, you went to the town library in fishnet stockings and heels stolen from your mothers' wardrobes; you barely made it through the door before the librarians asked to see your borrowing cards (which you dutifully handed over), and promptly called your parents to come remove you, your artistic intentions crushed.

That was the end of the photo shoots. But you'd caught the storytelling bug, you and Sarah, the vice that Hemingway says only death can stop. You wrote and illustrated Choose Your Own Adventure strips, in first one and then a series of identical red exercise books: the destined-to-be-legendary Red Book Choice Story, which one of you still owns in an attic somewhere. That book was pretty dangerous. In it you made good stuff happen to people you liked, the teachers who were kind and didn't throw chairs. You brought to life rumours of affairs and made the cool fifth formers fall in love with you. You gave the mean kids their comeuppance. It was secret, of course, until one day it wasn't. As stories went, it was a page-turner and it was gaining an underground reputation. Then Katie (not her real name) asked to read it. Katie was someone who took a persistent, vindictive delight in flipping up your netball skirt to reveal those blue regulation gym knickers and let's just say her narrative arc hadn't ended well. *Turn to page 48 to avenge the wrath of the schoolgirl demon.* Still, she scared you enough you didn't know how to refuse.

Here was the solution: you sat up all night to rewrite that book, the book that for months had demanded a more organic, fluid defiant kind of evolution. When you think of it now you wonder about the way you didn't stand up for the words. You want to believe this was what was needed to save the story (and your good-girl reputations), a mild, literary form of collateral damage, but this is not how it feels. Now it feels something closer to cowardice. Barthes says that the book creates meaning and then that meaning creates life. If so, then the meaning you were creating wasn't shitproof. One thing you don't know for certain; if it came to it, if you had to, how much would you really have risked to save that book? In this snow globe what you see is disappointing; two girls doing nothing but covering their steps.

But the thing about Choose Your Own Adventure is this: for every dead end, there is a way to renegotiate fate. A rope-bridge you didn't notice on page 61 leads you to safety across a gorge. As you are leaving the Forbidden Planet, some guy comes up to you. He taps your sleeve and asks, What are you after? Dylan Dog? Martin Mystery? And immediately you understand that he heard your conversation with the twitchy beards, that by some osmotic process he appreciates the vital nature of whatever it is you're trying to do. Here is your improbable reprieve, arriving like an angel with the correct vocabulary and everything.

You tell him you actually have no idea what you are after. It's a relief to confess it. You tell him the story of the comics in the septic tank. You tell him how you want to replace the shit-stained comics, the ones that never made it to safety in Sweden, which is where your friend ended up after the war. As you talk you realize how many gaps there are in what you know, what you're doing, but you learn this; strangers are so happy to help what they think of as a romantic (by which you mean old-school escapist, wild – and yes, crazy) notion. He pats you on the arm as if you're in need of Valium. Okay, he says. Okay.

The guy has a friend in Sarajevo who might be able to help. He takes your email address. The synchronicity buoys you up. It's like you're in a real comic book world of mystery and clues and leads. You don't say anything to your friend. You think you'll send him the comics for his birthday. It occurs to you that you don't know when his birthday is. Seriously, you don't have any idea what you are doing.

What part of the human brain compels it to see everything in relative terms? It doesn't even have to be the dramatic stuff. You understand how pattern finding has a deep, biological appeal. As soon as you heard the story of the comics in the septic tank, your own history became relative. You don't mean *less*. "The far becomes the near," says Rebecca Solnit. Things start to braid together in a new way; for a short time the only thing you could see, like a retina burn, was a teenage boy and his best friend sinking a plastic wrapped bundle of comics into a stinking shithole while on the other side of the continent a teenage girl and her best friend, both with a labyrinth-sized crush on David Bowie, repeat-pause VHS tapes on the dance scene where the Goblin King's crotch earns a credit all to itself.

About six years after the comics were hidden in the septic tank, you spent a summer working as an intern in the department of Prints and Drawings in the Musèe des Beaux Arts, Brussels. This was the summer you learned to eat again. You didn't know it was going to work this way, but standing in the great hall looking at Brueghel's Icarus, that all turned out to be part of the recovery.

W. H. Auden wrote a poem about that painting:

> About suffering they were never wrong
> the Old Masters. How well they understood
> its human position: how it takes place
> while someone else is eating or opening a window.

So many people saw your friend and his friend pushing a wheelbarrow of comic books around town, but even in war, everyone has somewhere to get to.

The sun shone as it had to, says Auden.

Perhaps one of the quiet tragedies of being human is that mostly, no-one is looking. They don't see something amazing. They see Icarus's legs disappearing into water and what they do is open a window. Here is what starts to get braided together then: the safety of your life and the danger in his, the way you were (not) eating or opening a window; the way he stuck two fingers up at that danger, leapt over the gate of a comic book collector in inner city Banja Luka and in defiance entered an adventure illustrated with invincible superheroes and big-busted apocalyptic monster women, a Promised Land. Icarus flying for the sun.

A few days later you hear from the Forbidden Planet guy's Sarajevo friend. Your emails muddle by in a mix of pretty bad English and rusty German, which is the best you can muster between you. He tells you that he has plenty of comics from the late 2000s, but anything from the 90s is impossible to get hold of; those books are like gold dust. You explain to him, in very general terms – because it's still hard to explain to yourself, to anyone, in complex terms – why it's important. Minutes pass. Wait a moment, he writes. Write you a new mail soon!

He gets back to you later that evening. You know these are not English language? he writes, as if things can't proceed until this has been established. These comics are in the Croatian language.

You ask if it's possible to get them in Bosnian. His reply is a series of bewildered exclamation marks and question marks and suddenly you realise a comic book is not just a comic book, that language is not just words uttered, that what you thought was knowledge is in fact just a haze, a silvered approximation of a war.

He sends you what appears to be a 1998 *Marti Misterija*, in Croatian, and says it's the best he can do, he can't get earlier. But he also has a whole bunch of Dylan Dogs and an Alan Ford, which is his personal favourite. He'll send those too. Registered fast packet, he says. *Important!* You lack the real words to show your gratitude, even though a tiny part of you is disappointed that you couldn't get what you really wanted, whatever that was. *Hvala* doesn't quite cut it. In English he writes that he has all (yes, all) the Martin Mystery series from the beginning to a few years ago when he stopped collecting. *There are not coming so many new . . .* he says and you feel the ache in the ellipsis. You don't ask why he stopped collecting. You are still thinking about the currency of these books. The way they might matter so much that a boy would put himself at risk to keep them safe, or that grown men would smuggle them to refugee camps. They must be fucking awesome, you think.

There's a giant eyeball on the cover of the 1998 Martin Mysterija. Inside, naked girls in some kind of swirling continuum. This MM is an art historian, adventurer, anthropologist and collector of unusual objects. *You had me at art historian!* you want to shout. A comic book hero who is part nerd! When they arrive, when you pore over them, in a language you can't read so you have to navigate through image alone, it is their ordinariness, the intimate, insular relationship they set up with their reader that really breaks your heart.

Only later do you realise what has been lost in translation – this is in fact a reissue, not as old as you thought. There are not coming so many new. A glacier shifts, the rope bridge breaks, and the path of this adventure comes to an end.

This much you know. What changes the world are the private wars people fight. Something amazing is the boys on the mountain, affording these stories of doomsdays and utopias the same status as diamonds and gold.

The war your father fought was in the air and it was public, and complicated. When your father returned from the Balkans he was a different man. Or maybe you were a different daughter and saw things you hadn't understood on his return from previous detachments: East Germany, Iraq. Lost, is the way you would describe him, Redrawn. Something your father heard in one town: a man had cut the head off his neighbour, a former friend, someone whose plants he had tended and whose dogs he had fed, and put it on a spike in his front garden. Above another town, a light attack aircraft was downed and the pilot ejected. He was found, mortally injured, by Ustaše Militia, who took him away, beat him to death and mutilated his already wounded body.

A week or so later your Sarajevo contact emails out of the blue to say he's been thinking. He might have something for you. He's actually got pretty much every comic out there, but he won't sell. What he will do is scan them and put some on DVD. Any ones you like.

There is something in this offer, this considered, delayed response, the desire to help flashed through with the desire to preserve the integrity of his collection at all costs, that makes you feel sad and simultaneously connected to something. Such generosity amongst an underground network of geeks. Your only tangible experience of Bosnia is this, comic books forming a chain out across, under, around Europe. Stories defying borders where people can't, people who will do whatever they must to restore the gaps in the narrative.

Once a semester you and your colleague Caron host an Open Mic Poetry night where you encourage your students to read and perform their own work. Some of them are a little bit afraid of poetry, but the camaraderie, the free wine and the craic fix that. You stand at the front of the lecture hall backlit by a PowerPoint that reads: *Words Have Power*. Words are smuggled from concentration camps, you tell them, through border posts, over mountains. Words are swallowed and remembered and burned into us in order that they survive. This is why we do what we do. This is why we write. This is why we read. Sometimes you worry whether this means anything to twenty-first-century teenagers whose biggest concerns, the media claim, involve thigh gaps and who their favourite celebrity is sleeping with. Then someone stands up, the quiet kid at the back who hasn't spoken yet, and reads about how his father is in prison for murdering his brother and you realise that it's not just the words that survive; we risk everything for them so that the strongest parts of ourselves will too.

That's how little I was afraid of being killed.

You're not sure if you believe him when he says this. But then, you know this to be true enough: on the only occasion you can say you were truly in grave and immediate danger of dying, you were pathologically practical. Half-mad with pain and morphine, you made arrangements with the theatre nurse, who humoured you by taking real notes, to cover your postgraduate dissertation supervision for a week. You told the anaesthetist that under no circumstances was he to have an argument with the surgeon over the afore-mentioned nurse if you went into VF, the way they did on the hospital shows. It's ok, he said, we're all happily married here. Then he pressed down on your windpipe to stop your stomach contents entering your lungs and put you under. You had no intention of dying, although the odds at the time were relatively high. You didn't even know what VF meant. What you're really saying is that maybe in the face of danger, we assume a hero's level of pragmatism, a clear ability to compartmentalise what is being risked away from what is needed, what is desired. It's possible this qualifies as a superpower.

You don't write back straight away to the Sarajevo guy. You're not quite sure what you'd be asking for. A DVD doesn't seem the same somehow. It's the tangible object, the restoration – the sheer materiality of your quest – that has been driving you, the book nerd's fantasy of the longed-for manuscript pressed into the outstretched hand. If you could travel to the afterlife and present Hemingway with a DVD of those stories from the suitcase stolen at the Gare de Lyon, you're pretty sure he would throw a daiquiri in your face.

The weather is turning cold here. One day your friend messages to tell you he wrote an essay on how to save comic books in time of war. He did it because you told him to. There's more to the story than what's in your snow globe. More than the wheelbarrow and the septic tank.

You're about to give an undergraduate writing class on constructing character. You're planning to do an exercise that draws on Tim O'Brien's story, "The Things They Carried," because you want your students to leave behind the trappings of their own autobiographies, just for a moment. Instead, at the very last minute, you ditch the schedule and tell them the true story of the boy who hid his comics in the septic tank. You watch your students' faces change as you talk. Even the two at the back who have been talking about the work they haven't done for their Renaissance Drama module are listening. Sharp winter light streams through the windows.

Even now you have not told your friend what you've been doing. Part of you is a little embarrassed. You experience what you come to think of as a distant cousin of survivor's guilt, but it's a superlative guilt that recycles and reactivates itself, guilty twice over – once for the simple fact that you didn't suffer his suffering, and again for its own fraudulent act of existing; this isn't even authentic, you survived nothing; it's survivor's guilt by proxy. Maybe this is your ouroboros come to get you. Damn it.

Still, in your tea break, you go back to your stuffy office and write your friend the pathetic story of how you tried and failed to hunt down his comics. You hesitate, just for a moment before pressing *send*. You're worried he will think badly of you, that he will think you stupid for believing that replacing a comic book might heal the other kinds of wound that war leaves a person with, the ones your friendship is too new, too distant to let you see, but the ones his fun stories about sad refugees tell you exist. That it could heal your own wounds, so small, so faraway in comparison. Or worse, that he will think you are appropriating what you're not entitled to, as if you are putting your hands under the skin of history, pressing on a bruise that isn't yours to feel.

What he really wanted – back then, now, both – was to be a comic book hero. You think about the ways to tell him he kind of already is.

Here is one way.

Tell him about the night the lonely girl, now a grown woman, hears the story of the comics for the first time. How she goes to sleep restless. How it feels as though her heart has been cut out, but in the morning she will wake to find it full and the restlessness renewed. Tell him how at first she thinks it's a kind of melancholia, but it's stranger and stronger than that. It is a teenage girl's breathless admiration for a teenage boy's bravado, combined with a mother's fear that any terrible thing that has ever happened to a child will now or in the future happen to her child. It is the concrete distillation of an abstract truth; that all the world's dark ugliness has never yet been able to extinguish that thing Nadine Gordimer calls the firefly flash of real life.

Tell him how that night the girl checked in on her son, as she does every night. How she saw in sleep little visible sign of the man he was slowly becoming. How it was hard not to compare him to the boy in the attic room in Bosnia, dreaming about his comics as they drift through raw sewage in their dark, plastic wombs. A little older than her son is now, true, but still a boy, just, whatever he'd probably say.

Don't tell him how she would cry for those shitty comic books she can't smell, because he wasn't crying over them and they were his comics. Explain instead that you will not forget this story of how once, two boys in Banja Luka did something brave and stupid and kind of miraculous. That miracles aren't always obvious. That miracles happen when someone is closing a window, or walking dully along. When it comes to it, really all you have to give is a story of a bungled comic book rescue, not the object restored. And it is a very small thing. Give it anyway. You may as well.

The first draft of "Everything I know about comic books* (*and what I am afraid to ask.)"

The following text is the very first draft Durneen sent to Mahmutović. It contains no edits or comments. Instead, this draft became a point of a conversation which is included after this text. That conversation shows the germination of the entire project which resulted in two essays, Durneen's "Everything I know about comic books* (*and what I am afraid to ask.)" and Mahmutović's "How to Save Comics in Times of War".[1] It is about the nuts and bolts of the storytelling as well as the very content of the essay that lead to the second draft, which Mahmutović edited (displayed immediately after the conversation). Our intention with this text is to show the readers a more complex process of editing that is not about mere tweaking of the finished text, but goes deeper into the process of the creation of a story.

> Everything begins in
> *The Ordinary World.*

In the summer of 1992, or thereabouts, a seventeen-year-old boy and his best friend filled a wheelbarrow with comics, heaved it through the woods above the Bosnian town of Banja Luka and looked out a hiding place for their stash of Druuna and Silver Surfers. They just couldn't get enough of these comics, imported from England and Italy and America. The boy really wanted to be a comic book hero. To begin with, that's the most important thing you need to know. That's why one way to tell this story is through the oldest kind of story, the monomyth. *A hero ventures forth from the world of the common day into a region of supernatural wonder.* The world the boy was living in was not especially ordinary anymore, but not everything gets worse. Nothing, the boy felt, beat the wonders of reading comics in wartime.

In the summer of 1992 an almost-fifteen-year-old girl and her best friend went to the annual Strawberry Fair in Cambridge, England. The girl thought maybe they would ride the waltzer and pretend to drink lemon Hooch with the kids she hoped might stop giving her a hard time if she acted a little more like them. Instead, outside

---

1 The two essays were published head to head as one larger, hybrid piece in *World Literature Today* in 2015, and in 2016 adapted and broadcast on BBC Radio 4.

a dirty canvas tent, they found a bucket of goldfish waiting to be transferred to the cellophane globes hanging off the nearby Hook a Duck stand. The fish looked sad, a seething mass of orange like a solar explosion in a plastic tub. The girl and her friend looked around, picked up the unattended bucket and walked fast until they were two streets away from the fair, suddenly in charge of hundreds of bright, starry fish, water surging over the bucket's lip at every step and soaking the toes of their Doc Marten 8-holes.

The boy and his friend had been slipping across military checkpoints to grow their collection for some months. Now the need to hide the comic books from the soldiers was more pressing. They were not afraid, although they should have been. Others were burying necklaces and gold; the boy and his friend were trying to hide stories, entire worlds. They considered these stories worth dying for. This meant there were also people who considered them worth killing for.

They rejected the woods on the grounds of wild animals. So they pushed that wheelbarrow through the town, looking all over for a better place, a safer place, somewhere they might come back to once the war was over – someplace that might still exist in spite of violent effort to redraw the country, to change its contours. The boy devised a cunning plan. He wrapped the comics in plastic bags and lowered them into a septic tank, reasoning that you'd have to be pretty determined to look for contraband there. The boy was not afraid of the soldiers, but after a while he grew pretty worried maybe those plastic bags weren't actually quite so shitproof. He tossed and turned in bed for weeks thinking about his comics. He wanted to read them, wanted them so badly it was a kind of desire, burning at him, nudging into his sleep. It occurred to him that *coming back* meant first they had to leave, and they were still here. It occurred to him that before that time to return came, the comic books might dissolve or worse, whatever worse might be.

The girl was kind of lonely. She read a lot. Too much, maybe. The other girls in her class were pretty and were learning how to kiss the boys in the dark of the school drama theatre. The boys in her class called her a nerd and made vomiting sounds when they played spin the bottle and the bottle stopped on her. Somewhere around the beginning of 1992 she had decided to stop eating, as if that might make a difference. As if loneliness and food were directly connected somehow and you could fix one by rationing the other.

The boy's intuition was spot on. What hit him when he went back to the septic tank to retrieve the comics was a damp, ripe smell, the smell of human shit and trees, which of all things is actually just the smell of life. They no longer had that supple, smoky scent of ink and wood pulp, the vanillin warmth of ancient paper, but it would not make him love the comic books any less. Maybe this evidence of the struggle they had been through even made him love them a little more.

The girl smelled of White Musk perfume from the Body Shop, like every other fourteen-year-old girl in Western Europe, and possibly faintly of white cabbage, of which she was eating a disproportionate amount. She watched Tintin on Sunday mornings and scared herself with Twilight Zone and that was as much as she knew about comic books. By the summer of 1992 she hadn't eaten anything except cabbage cooked in vegetable stock for nearly four months. She had a crush on Cyrano de Bergerac. Partly this was because of Gerard Depardieu, who hadn't yet gotten fat and started pissing in planes, but partly because she still half-believed in the existence of heroes that didn't look like heroes, the ones that maybe were OK about it if you got good grades and wrote poems and didn't have big boobs or straight teeth.

The boy used up all his mother's expensive deodorant to take away the smell of shit-stained comic book paper from his attic bedroom. His mother wanted to kill him. His words.

One time the girl's mother threw a plate of food at her. Why can't you just be normal? the mother shouted, and she really wanted to know. The girl's father was in the business of reconnaissance. She hadn't seen him for some months. In summer 1992 she didn't actually know where he was, other than that a war in a place that was no longer Yugoslavia had taken him away.

Not long after this the boy became a refugee. Some of the comic books made it onto the buses with him, bound for Sweden, the bright green northern lights, safety. The others – I have not asked what happened to them.

Eventually, officially, wars come to an end. Some people get to go back home, like the girl's father. Mostly war follows you, invisibly, internally. You can make it your business to study the writing of war, but there is always the knowledge, a deep guilt in the regolith of you, that no matter how much you read you can never, actually, know. Lives converge until the moment they absolutely don't.

The boy and the girl grew up and found themselves becoming adults on different sides of a changed continent, one in a city of islands under the Midnight Sun, the other on the south coast of Cornwall where the tourists don't bother to go. They both became writers. The boy wrote about the war. The girl wrote about being lonely. They both became parents. By 2014 they had children not much younger than they had been back in the summer of 1992.

They both went to Vienna to talk about short stories. The girl learned about the concept of manifest yearning. The boy read to hushed audiences of that long journey north from Banja Luka and caused a stampede for the only copy of his book of fun stories about sad refugees. It turned out they both were a little in love with Hemingway, which is a good way to start talking to someone. What this all meant was that one night some months later, after they returned to their respective homes and had got past the stage of asking each other the way to the beach in loud voices, the boy, now a man, wrote to the girl, now a woman, and more than twenty years after it originally happened, told her the story of the comic books hidden in the septic tank and broke her heart.

The call to adventure

This can happen without you knowing. The night the girl hears the story of the comic books for the first time, she goes to sleep restless. If it feels as though her heart has been cut out, in the morning – like the plant in the desert found by

Ondaatje's English Patient – she will wake to find it full and the restlessness renewed. When it comes, the sudden thump of this heartbreak has no shape, no choreography. It's entire. It is old. It comes at her like the roar of some distant wild animal. 'It'. She doesn't know what 'it' is. At first she thinks it's a kind of melancholia, but it's not, it's stranger and stronger than that. Here is one way to describe it: it is a teenage girl's breathless admiration for a teenage boy's valiant bravado, combined with a mother's fear that any terrible thing that has ever happened to a child will now or in the future happen to her child. It is the concrete distillation of an abstract truth; that all the world's dark ugliness has never yet been able to stop the firefly flash of real life. She can't quite hear the words of it yet, but something is calling, yes.

She checks in on her son. His face is soft; in sleep there is little visible sign of the man he is slowly becoming. She thinks of her friend in his attic room, dreaming about his comics as they drift through raw sewage in their dark, plastic wombs. A little older than her son is now, true, but still a boy, just, whatever he'd probably say. She would cry for those shitty comic books she can't smell, only that seems wrong because he wasn't crying over them and they were his comics. For those books, he would stake his life. *You crazy, brave boy,* she thinks, which in her head are the words that sound like crying feels.

* * *

Actually, the hero is first supposed to refuse the call to adventure. I tell my friend, the writer, the boy, Adnan, that he has to write about this – an essay on how to save comic books in time of war.

I was really stupid, wasn't I? he asks.
No, I say, and it's not entirely a lie. It's what Indiana Jones would do.
That's how little I was worried about being killed, he says. Bloody geek.
But geeks are so much cooler than nerds.
What?
Sorry. I thought that was my inside voice.

My eldest son is a proud Doctor Who geek, and inordinately fond of that viral song "Dumb Ways to Die." He worries a lot about being killed. By solar flare, freak asteroid impact, zombie apocalypse, Ebola. I try to imagine him avoiding soldiers and navigating checkpoints, hiding anything or even understanding that he might need to, and remember how last time he made lunch for himself he used a tea strainer to drain a can of tuna fish. It's pretty unlikely the odds would be in his favour

I wonder what part of our brain compels us to see everything in relative terms. It doesn't even have to be the dramatic stuff. *You were doing this while I was* – Pattern finding has a deep, biological appeal. As soon as I heard the story of the comics in the septic tank, my own history became relative. I don't mean *less*. It's just that things start to braid together in a new way; for a short time the only thing I could see, like a retina burn, was a teenage boy and his best friend sinking a plastic wrapped bundle of comic books into a stinking shithole while on the other side of the continent a teenage girl and her best friend, both with a labyrinth-sized crush on David Bowie, repeat-pause VHS tapes on the dance scene where the Goblin King's crotch earns a credit all to itself.

About six years after the comic books were hidden in the septic tank I spent a summer working as an intern in department of Prints and Drawings in the *Musèe des Beaux Arts*, Brussels. This was the summer I learned to eat again. I didn't know it was going to work this way, but standing in the great hall looking at Brueghel's Icarus, the amazing boy who fell from the sky while a *ship sailed calmly on* – that all turned out to be part of the recovery.

W. H. Auden wrote a poem about that painting: 'About suffering they were never wrong/the Old Masters. How well they understood/ its human position: how it takes place/while someone else is eating or opening a window.' I wonder if this is the part that moves me the most about Adnan's story. There were lots of people who saw him and his friend Armin pushing a wheelbarrow of comic books around town, but even in war, everyone has somewhere to get to. *The sun shone as it had to*, says Auden. Perhaps this invisibility is what protected them, what stopped them getting into the kind of trouble I can barely imagine. Or perhaps one of the quiet tragedies of being human is that we know fine well how everything is relative, but also that mostly, no-one is looking. We don't see something amazing. We see Icarus's legs disappearing into water and what we do is open a window.

Here is what gets braided together, then; the safety of my life and the way I was (not) eating or opening a window and the danger in his, the way he stuck two fingers up at it, leapt over the gate of a comic book collector in inner city Banja Luka and in defiance, entered an adventure illustrated with invincible superheroes and big-busted apocalyptic monster women, a promised land; Icarus flying for the sun.

Supernatural aid

Which is what the monomyth promises as a means of help from without – maps or weaponry or a kind of magic talisman, maybe. This is apparently how every story that has ever been told proceeds. This is how things change. Something to help the hero face the challenges ahead.

How can I explain this? Sometimes you just have to say things even if they make no sense. It's like I am watching the scene from somewhere far off, from above, these two kids and their wheelbarrow, going up one street and down another, their frustration (and perhaps also their fear) growing, although Adnan never mentions that. It's like seeing the whole thing through a snow globe. Asimov's chronoscope. Vonnegut would call it slipping in time.

The urge to *do* something is visceral, it starts somewhere in my throat and rises. If I could shout down through the time vortex. If he could look up into the swirling cogs/ether/matrix to see me waving. What would I say? Throw me your comics, I'll keep them safe for you? Or – hang on, I'm coming down, let me help push the damn wheelbarrow? A girl, I think, especially a nerdy one, might have come up with a better plan than a septic tank. If a comic book could change history, I think. And, what does that even mean?

It's not like I don't know how time travel works. The rules, that is. I've read Brian Cox's $E=MC^2$ more than once and am still not entirely sure about the analogy of the very fast train – the quantum bit. But everyone knows you cannot change points in a timeline, not without having catastrophic consequences for humanity. The flutter of pages in 1992 creates a tsunami on the other side of space and time.

Still. The things a comic book might be able to do.

We don't actually mention the comic book essay again for a while. Adnan sends me a different essay to proof-read, this one is about faith and forgiveness. Here I see he's ambivalent about forgiving a person who once stole his Bonelli comics. He's joking, sure, but – those comic books again, I think. They really do mean something, huh?

I read the essay about ten times. I want to ask so many things. Bonelli. *Bonelli*. I commit it to memory. Italian. Were these the comics sunk into the septic tank and ravaged by shit and expensive deodorant? I don't know. I think of that story about Hadley Hemingway, the famous one in which she catches a train to visit Ernest in Lausanne and whilst waiting at the Gare de Lyon her suitcase containing every last one of the original Nick Adams stories is stolen. I imagine the despair of knowing that there is nothing to replace the thing you have lost, an emptiness that stretches out about as long as the journey to Switzerland.

An idea comes to me – a crazy one, I see that right from the outset. It comes at me the way anything obvious and also impossible arrives in your mind. I want to replace those ruined comics. Don't ask me why.

Crossing the threshold

Here's the real problem. I know nothing about comic books. But I work alongside magical agents and allies; people who actually do. I leave behind the sleek contemporary corridors of the university in which I teach and cross over to the Victorian halls of the Cambridge School of Art. But although there are geeks, collectors, and experts on graphic literature in every room, this one seems out of even their league. Someone knows someone somewhere in Slovenia who maybe once had a thing about comic books. Will that help?

It doesn't. I go commercial. I try that other bastion of geekdom, Forbidden Planet on Burleigh Street, the new, improved store that makes a lot of promises about being the world's number one for your comic book needs. My plan is to look like I know what I'm doing – because isn't that what Indiana Jones would do? So when I ask for help in tracking down early 90s Bonelli from the former Yugoslavia I assume a kind of casual, professional air as though I do this all the time. *No time for love, Doctor Jones.*

The assistants at the counter look at me like I'm mad. Their beards twitch. Wouldn't Marvel or DC be good enough? they want to know. The word I have fixed on is

Bonelli, so I shake my head as if I'm disappointed by *their* lack of knowledge. It has to be early 90s. It has to be from – I find myself getting tangled up in the geography. The Balkans, I say in the end. But as I'm leaving, the IT guy, behind the desk to fix some system or other, comes up to me and pulls my sleeve before I walk out of the door. What are you after? he says. Dylan Dog? Martin Mystère? I don't know, I tell him. It's a relief to confess it. I tell the IT guy the story of the comic books in the septic tank. I tell him how I want to replace the shit-stained comics. The lost comics, the ones that never made it to Sweden. As I talk I realize how many gaps there are in what I know, what I'm doing, but here is what I learn; strangers are so happy to help what they think of as a romantic (by which I mean old-school escapist, wild – and yes, crazy) notion. He pats me on the arm as if I'm in need of something. Okay, he says. Okay.

The IT guy has a friend in Sarajevo who might be able to help. He takes my email address. What are the odds, I think? The synchronicity buoys me up. It's like another world has opened in front of me, a (secret) mission, a real comic book world of mystery and clues and leads. I don't say anything to Adnan. I have the idea maybe I'll send him the comic books for his birthday. I don't actually know when his birthday is. Seriously, I don't have any idea what I am doing.

Challenges and temptations

I said I know nothing about comic books. This is mostly, but not entirely, true – it's just that we're not talking your Silver Surfer or Blueberry. We're definitely not talking Corto Maltese. My friend Sarah and I were avid devotees of the *Just Seventeen* photo story. Our dream was to make one of our own and sell it to the magazine, get a regular segment maybe. We were not seventeen and we hadn't even kissed a boy, but this did not stop us spending hours devising storylines, longer still staging the photographs themselves. Our inspiration was drawn largely from an improbable mix of *Wuthering Heights*, *Neighbours* and those Virginia Andrews books that all the girls were passing around school in paper bags. On one occasion, planning a surreptitious photo shoot, we went to the town library in stockings and heels stolen from our mothers' wardrobes; we barely made it through the door before the librarians asked to see our borrowing cards (which we dutifully handed over) and promptly called our parents to remove us.

That brought the photo shoots to an abrupt end. But Sarah and I had an alternative outlet for our creative endeavours. We were addicted to Choose Your Own Adventures and wrote and illustrated our own, in first one and then a series of identical red exercise books: the destined-to-be-legendary Red Book Choice Story, which one of us still owns in an attic somewhere. The book was pretty dangerous, it was fair to say. In it we made good stuff happen to people we liked, teachers who were nice to us. We brought to life rumours of affairs and made the cool fifth formers fall in love with us. We gave the kids who were mean to us what could euphemistically be called their comeuppance. It was secret, of course, until one day it wasn't. As stories went, it was a page-turner and it was gaining an underground reputation.

Then one girl, a girl who took great delight in pulling my hair and flipping up my netball skirt to reveal those stupid, enormous blue gym knickers, asked to read it. Let's just say her narrative arc hadn't ended well. Still, she scared me enough that I didn't know how to refuse.

I sat up all night to rewrite that book, the book that had taken months to evolve organically, defiantly, into a complex web of fantasies fulfilled and thwarted, ideal lives created and lived. When I think of it now I wonder about the way I didn't stand up for the words, that when faced with a test I chose to betray the truths they were supposed to expose. I want to believe that was what was needed to save the story, (and our good-girl reputations; no doubt we would have faced an indeterminate number of detentions had the teachers found it) – a kind of mild, literary collateral damage – but this is not how it feels. Now it feels like cowardice. Barthes says that the book creates meaning and then that meaning creates life. If so, then the meaning I was creating was fraudulent, the life a lie. One thing I am ashamed that I don't know for certain; how much would I have risked to save that book, any book, in time of war, if in peacetime I was too afraid to stand up and be counted?

A few days later I hear from the IT guy's Sarajevo friend. Our emails muddle by in a mix of pretty bad English and rusty German, which is the best we can muster between us. He tells me that he has plenty of comics from the late 2000s, but anything from the 90s is impossible to get hold of; those books are like gold dust. I explain to him, in very general terms (because I am having trouble explaining, to myself, to anyone, in complex terms) why it's important to me. Minutes pass. Wait a moment, he types. Write you a new mail!

He gets back to me later that evening. You know these are not English language, don't you? he says, as if we can't proceed until this has been established. These comics are in Croatian language.

I ask him if it's possible to get them in Bosnian. His reply is a series of exclamation and question marks and suddenly I realise how a comic book is not just a comic book, how language is not just lexis, how little I understand – really understand – of that whole conflict given I don't even know something fundamental like what language my friend would read his Dylan Dog in, not for sure.

The Sarajevo guy sends me a 1998 *Marti Misterija*, in Croatian, and says it's the best he can do, he can't get earlier. But he also has a whole bunch of Dylan Dogs and an Alan Ford, which is his personal favourite. He'll send those too. Registered fast packet, he says. *Important!* I lack the real words to show my gratitude, even though a tiny part of me is disappointed that I couldn't get what I really wanted, whatever that was. *Hvala* doesn't quite cut it. In English he writes that he has all (yes, all) the Martin Mystère series from the beginning to a few years ago when he stopped collecting. There are not coming so many new . . . he says and I feel the true sadness in the ellipsis. I don't ask him why he stopped collecting. I am still thinking about the currency of these books. The way they might matter so much that a boy would put himself at risk to keep them safe, or that grown men would smuggle them to refugee camps. They must be fucking awesome, I think.

When they arrive, when I pore over them – in a language I can't read so I am navigating through image alone – it is their ordinariness, the intimate, insular relationship they set up with their reader, that really breaks my heart. There's a giant eyeball on the cover of the 1998 Martin Mystère. Inside, naked girls in some kind of swirling continuum. Martin Mystère – Mystery in America, Misterija in Croatia, Marma Manithan Martin in South India – is an art historian, adventurer, anthropologist and collector of unusual objects. *You had me at art historian!* I want to shout. A comic book hero who is part nerd! It's not important that I understand exactly. I look at the comics and what I feel is that same thrill of discovery, of finding an entire universe world to inhabit. It's the way reading makes you feel alive; not in the way that is the opposite of death but real and present, there and nowhere else but *there*.

This much I know. The things that might change the world are the private wars we fight. The deals we make with ourselves as to how far we'd go for something we love. The something amazing is the strength and power and purpose in what those boys did up on the mountain, affording these stories of doomsday and utopias that they tried to bury the same status as diamonds and gold.

Abyss

There are some things Adnan and I have not talked about. The things he does not say in the story of the comic books in the septic tank.

When my father returned from the Balkans he was a different man. Or maybe I was a different daughter and saw things I hadn't understood on his return from previous detachments; East Germany, Iraq. Bewildered, is the way I would describe him. Traumatized, yes. Something my father had heard in one town: A man had cut the head off his neighbour, a former friend, someone whose plants he had tended and whose dogs he had fed, and put it on a spike in his front garden. Above another town, a light attack aircraft was downed and the pilot ejected. He was found, mortally injured, by Ustaŝe Militia, who took him away, beat him to death and mutilated his already wounded body.

Adnan tells me one day about an old television monologue, the story of a peasant who goes to Austria to work. The peasant meets this man who tells him there's no such country as Bosnia.

No matter what the narrator says, Adnan tells me, the man stubbornly refuses all arguments, so the narrator gets so pissed he leaves the good life and goes back to his village out of spite. It's so funny.

What happens when he gets back to his village, I ask, trying to imagine how it is funny when it sounds so sad.

The story ends. He walks down the hill, heavily gesticulating. Repeating the words angrily, 'and he tells ME there's no Bosnia'.

Death and rebirth

A week or so later my Sarajevo contact emails me out of the blue to say he's been thinking. He might have something for me. He's actually got pretty much every comic out there, but he won't sell. But what he will do is scan them for me and put some on DVD. Any ones I like. There is something in this offer, this considered, delayed response, the desire to help flashed through with the desire to preserve the integrity of his collection at all costs, that makes me feel sad and simultaneously connected to something. Such generosity amongst an underground network of geeks. I think of the comic books forming a chain out across, under, around Europe and how those who know will go out of their way to restore the gaps in the narrative.

Once a semester my colleague Caron and I host an Open Mic Poetry night where we encourage our students to read and perform their own work alongside us. They are all afraid of poetry, but they like the camaraderie, the free wine and the craic. We stand at the front of the lecture hall backlit by a PowerPoint that reads *Words Matter*. Words are smuggled from concentration camps, we tell them, through border posts, over mountains. Words are swallowed and remembered and burned into us in order that they survive. This is why we do what we do. This is why we write. This is why we read. Sometimes you wonder if this means anything to twenty-first-century teenagers whose biggest concerns involve thigh gaps and who their favourite celebrity is sleeping with. Then someone stands up, the quiet girl at the back who hasn't spoken yet, and reads about recovering from sexual abuse and you realise that it's not just the words that survive; we risk everything for them so that the strongest parts of ourselves will too.

That's how little he was afraid of being killed. I'm not sure if I believe Adnan when he says this. But then, I know this to be true enough: on the only occasion I can say I was truly in grave and immediate danger of dying, I was surprisingly, pathologically, practical. Half-mad with pain and morphine, I made arrangements with the theatre nurse, who humoured me by taking real notes, to cover my postgraduate dissertation supervision for a week. I told the anaesthetist that under no circumstances was he to have an argument with the surgeon over the afore-mentioned nurse if I went into VF, the way they did on the hospital shows. It's ok, he told me, we're all happily married here. Then he pressed down on my windpipe to stop my stomach contents entering my lungs and put me under/shut me up. I had no intention of actually dying, although the odds at the time were relatively high. I didn't even know what VF meant.

I think what I'm really saying is that maybe in the face of true danger, we assume a hero's level of pragmatism, a clear ability to compartmentalise what we're risking away from what we need, what we desire. It's possible this qualifies as a superpower, awesome in the real sense of the word; life-affirming.

I don't write back straight away to the IT guy's friend in Sarajevo. I'm not quite sure what I'd be asking for. A DVD doesn't seem quite the same somehow. It's the tangible object, the restoration – the sheer materiality of the quest – that has been driving me, the book nerd's fantasy of the longed-for manuscript pressed into the outstretched hand. If I could travel to the afterlife and present Hemingway with a DVD of those stories from the suitcase stolen at the Gare de Lyon, I'm pretty sure he would throw a daiquiri in my face.

The reward, seizing the sword

In most definitions of the hero's journey, the ultimate boon is the achievement of the quest. I can't offer it, seeing as I couldn't achieve it, not fully. It's also not entirely my quest. It's a quest I took the hero on without telling him, which probably breaks all the rules. Still, I'm a writer. I can make my own narrative. I can travel in time whenever I want, if it comes to it. Here's one way I would end the quest, if I could.

I see myself, an older (by which I mean earlier) me, not quite fifteen, awkward and nerdy and leaning into the vortex that is open and waiting for this moment, this one moment, above a weirdly perfumed attic bedroom in Banja Luka, shouting down to the seventeen-year-old Adnan. I'm sorry, I would shout. This is the best I could do. I hope it's a good one! And then I would throw down the book, Marti Misterija – no, sorry, pass, he would kill me for throwing it. The most important comic book in all of history.

At the very least he would look puzzled, I am sure. It's 1992 for a start and there's no way of knowing how those big-breasted girls are going to get into the river in six years' time. Never mind that there's a crazy English girl opening up time and space to give him a comic book.

You only get a minute in these situations. Anything more tears the fabric of reality apart. So I haven't got long. If I had only a minute to say anything, I would say this. *By the way*, I would say as the time mists start to whirl back in – and it is not as an afterthought, but as the first thing I thought. *By the way*, I think what you did was really *fenomenalan*. Saving your books. That's, like, the bravest thing ever.

Cool. Hvala, he would say back, looking tough, like he didn't really care what I thought, like people said that kind of thing to him all the time.

There are other versions. But this is the one I'm going with here.

Transformation, the road back

The weather is turning cold here. One day my friend messages to tell me his essay, the real essay on how to save comic books in time of war, is finished. I'm about to give an undergraduate writing class on constructing character. I'm planning to do an exercise that draws on Tim O'Brien's story, 'The Things They Carried'; I want my students to think about the things we don't show the world, the ones that define character from within. I want them to leave behind the trappings of their own autobiographies. Instead, at the very last minute, I ditch my schedule and tell my students the true story of the boy who hid his comics in the septic tank. The things we risk our life for. I watch my students' faces change as I talk. I have their complete attention, all of them, even the two at the back who have been talking about the work they haven't done for their Renaissance Drama module. The words break in my mouth like they are tiny spears of porcelain. We all sit quietly with the sharp winter light streaming through the windows.

Even now I have not told Adnan what I've been doing. Part of me is a little embarrassed, by the intensity of how I feel, the way I suspect I have no right to feel it the way I do. I experience what I come to think of as a distant cousin of survivor's guilt, but it's a superlative guilt that recycles and reactivates itself, guilty twice over – once for the simple fact that I didn't suffer his suffering, and again for its own fraudulent act of existing; this isn't even authentic, I survived nothing; it's survivor's guilt by proxy. My students are obsessed by the idea of ouroboros, something chasing its own tail. Maybe this is my ouroboros come to get me, I think. Damn it.

In my tea break I go back to my stuffy office and write him, without stopping, the pathetic story of how I tried and failed to hunt down the comic books that may or may not have been destroyed during, or after, their meeting with the septic tank. Most probably the comics I have been chasing were never there. I hesitate before pressing *send* because I am worried he will think badly of me. I'm worried that he will think I'm dumb for believing that replacing a comic book might heal the other kinds of wound that war leaves a person with, the ones our friendship is too new, too distant to let me see, but the ones his fun-sad stories tell me exist. Or worse, that he will know I have only an outsider's perspective and will think I am romanticising something, appropriating what I am not entitled to.

What I really want to do is explain that as long as I live I will not forget this story of how, once, two boys in Banja Luka did something brave and stupid and, yes, miraculous. Awesome.

The return with elixir

I finish my message. I do press send. What it comes to it this really is all I have to give – my story of the failed comic book rescue, not the book itself – not the object restored, and it is a very small thing. No magic elixir. I just want him to know that I can see it, the boys on the mountain with their wheelbarrow, the way they are splashing their trousers with sewage as they fish the Silver Surfer out of the septic tank. What I see might be inaccurate, caught only in relief like a magic lantern show, but it's visible. I'm trying to say, now I understand that nothing beats reading comics in wartime anyway.

And this I know too: my friend does not need, or even want me to move time and space for him, to find his lost books. Some things stay lost. Not every gap in history can be filled. *The hero is the champion of things becoming, not of things become.* Maybe that itself is a different kind of elixir.

What he really wanted, still does, was to be a comic book hero. I contemplate how to tell him he kind of already is. But this I do not say in the message I send. I'll tell him that some other time.

Writing in response
Chat between Lucy Durneen and Adnan Mahmutović

The following exchange took place in November 2014. The conversation, although it includes reflections on Mahmutovic´'s essay, is here meant to give insight into the shaping of Durneen's work. The conversation took place on Facebook Messenger and was later followed by extensive writing, rewriting, and editing of Durneen's story.

Durneen

I've been thinking a lot about comics over the last few weeks – something I don't know a huge amount about, I have to say. But what I do know is that as long as I live I will not forget (as in, Alzheimer's will have to take it from me) the story of the boy hiding his comics in a septic tank. It's the fearlessness that I can't shake off. How much those comics meant to you. The image comes to me in the strangest ways, like I am slipping in time, as Vonnegut would say. It's like I can see you, with the wheelbarrow of comics, but I can't touch, I can't move or intervene. It's like I'm watching the whole thing through a snow globe. It breaks my heart. If a comic book could change time, I find myself thinking.

I read your essay. I read it like ten times. I had this rather pathetic idea, I would find you a comic. Bonelli, right? It becomes like a (secret) mission. It's like another world has opened up to me, a proper comic book world of mystery and clues and leads. I realise I know nothing and I have no idea where to start so I go to Forbidden Planet in Cambridge and ask for help in tracking down early 90s Bonelli from the former Yugoslavia. They look at me like I'm mad, but as I'm leaving, the IT guy who has come to fix some system or other comes up to me and says he has a friend in Sarajevo who might be able to help.

So I hear from the friend. He tells me that he has plenty of comics from the late 2000s, but anything from the 90s is impossible to get hold of, they're like gold dust. I explain to him, in very general terms, why it's important to me. He gets back to me later that evening. You do know these won't be in English, don't you? he says. I ask him if it's possible to get them in Bosnian. His reply is a series of exclamation and question marks and suddenly I realise how a comic book is not just a comic, how language is not just words, how little I understand – really understand – of a conflict that I watched on the news and discussed at school but I don't even know something simple like what language you would read your comics in. The Sarajevo guy sends me a 1998 Martin Mysterre, in Croatian, and says it's the best he can do, he can't get earlier. I think, I want to send this to you for your birthday, but you don't want a birthday present and anyway, would it make you happy – or sad, or angry, even? I can't stop thinking about the power of these comics. Their currency. The way they might matter so much that a boy would put himself at risk to keep them safe.

A week or so later the guy contacts me to say he's actually got pretty much every comic out there, but he won't sell. What he will do is scan them for me and put some on DVD. Any ones I like. There is something in this offer, this considered response, that makes me feel sad and simultaneously connected to something. I haven't written back yet. What would I even be asking for? But I just wanted to tell you about it. And I have this 1998 comic for you, if you would like it.

Mahmutović

Lucy, this is crazy. This story of you hunting down comics is equally and even more poignant than my story about septic tank. (I'll send you that soon.)

Bonelli is an Italian publisher and they mostly produced pulp. Martin Mystery is one of those series, sort of Indiana Jones only with a nerd main character. I enjoyed them as a kid, but the ones that stay with me are the more grown-up stories. Franco Belgian school produced more of those quality books than the Italians. That's why few Bonelli pulp fictions can be found in English. Lately they translated som Dylan Dog series. So you don't need to find me a comic that old, though I'll take that MM from 98. Seriously. The thought counts more than anything, but seriously, if you wrote a story, an essay really, about this, using the material you just wrote in this message, that'd be an amazing complementary story to mine. It'd be so damn cool to publish both in the same journal.

Durneen

He sent me some of those too. I have a whole box of comics I can't read from a random guy. Dylan Dog, I mean.

Mahmutović

I'll send you some good comics. Do you have an iPad or some tablet? If not, you can also read some off computer screen.

Durneen

Love that idea of a complementary essay thing. In seminar break, more later. Not sure how to do it though. How to "form" it. Will think.

Mahmutović

You have half of it written in your message. Here's a draft of my essay. Not terribly long but compact, I hope.

Durneen

Just leaving work, going to read on bus. So cold! It's like winter just arrived today. Am also on the case with the novel WIP ... Slight distraction as my dear son just informed me he has to make a volcano cake for geography (?!) ... Which means basically I am now making a volcano cake for geography. It's ok though, I figured it out. Cupcakes, each with a little fondant volcano, Etna, Vesuvius, Krakatoa ...

Mahmutović

Great. Thanks.

Durneen

Oh ... So funny and sad and beautiful... But you know you would probably have had more luck with the mercy fuck if you had not been reading so many comics, right? Seriously though ... I love the way it's so moving, but also upbeat. Very real. And the compactness works for it.

Mahmutović

Back then I never heard of the concept of a mercy fuck. Besides, no girl could live up to Druuna, right? Bloody geek. Good luck with the volcanos.

And, do you think you could do a piece related to this. I'm really moved by the whole thing. Never seen or heard anything like that. Amazing.

Durneen

Yep, I'm going to try ... but it will be nowhere near as good as yours. How do you think it should work as a companion piece? Consciously? Or like I never read yours? I have two days off now, so am going to start on it after the bloody volcanos.

And I have never been moved by anything as much as you telling me about the comics in the first place.

I have to tell my friend Tiffani about the Druuna. She's researching monster sex for her PhD. I'm not even joking.

Mahmutović

I'm thinking unconsciously, at first. Starting with me telling you about the event, and you telling me to write an essay about it, and then you do that other stuff behind my back, and then the two stories converge.

PhD on monster sex? Who's paying for it, I'd like to write my second PhD. I haven't read these since I was kid. He has other stuff too, but Druuna and new erotica made him most money I think.

Durneen

Ok. I'm done. But I'm just checking some stuff. I just want to be sure – what year did you hide the comic books? I was trying to go back through these messages but it turns out there's like 3000 of them. I think you said you were 17? Just don't want to get stuff wrong.

Mahmutović

In 1992.

Durneen

Ok, that's what I have. Right. I think I can send you it then. I'm so nervous about sending you this. It became longer than I thought, too long, but it's ok, another draft can do some brutal cuts on it – I just thought I would send what it turned out to be for now. I've not written anything like this before. It was harder than I thought it would be – in the end, I took the advice of Gertrude Stein to Picasso when he was struggling to paint her portrait – "paint me out and then paint me in when I'm not here." I had to think you weren't there so I could paint you in, and now that's done, I can cut it down, take stuff out, whatever.

Now I need to eat. I didn't stop writing all day and now I'm ravenous. Meat! Where's the meat . . .

Mahmutović

Thank you. Fenomenalno. I have some ideas for the next draft it's ok. "If" it's ok. Loved getting to know you. Nerd? Ha.

Durneen

Oh yeah. SUCH a nerd. And it's yours now – whatever you want to do for the next draft . . . just say and I'll do it.

Mahmutović

This is your story and though its related to me, it is about you. So to begin with I think there is too much me, too much of my story. Your essay is best when I'm just a hint in the background. I think you should start with you hunting down comics in Sarajevo and work your way back and forth through time.

This is not a linear story. So the reader wonders why is she doing this. Thing is, you have so many details from my essay and yet those were not a part of this journey. Just that image of the septic tank.

Durneen

Interesting, because to start with, in the earlier draft, I was worried there was too much me and not enough of your story. But then I was also conscious that your story was not *my* story, so I kind of switched it.

Mahmutović

I was writing on the phone on the way to work so lots of weird typos.

Yes, the story may be centering around this thing I told you, but it's about you. I'd begin with the scene when you're going to the store, because it shows so much about your character, and then unfold. Linearity takes away something from the entire thing.

Imagine that snowball and the story is you drifting in and out of it, reaching in and pulling out.

Durneen

Ok, snowballing . . . right. And so from the store I unfold . . . Where? Back to the original story of the septic tank? Or somewhere else? On my way to work too so may disappear at some point. Teaching until 6.

Mahmutović

Just finished my class on editing here. I'm not sure what's best to go into next, in terms of scenes. Let me reread it and see.

But at this point, does this make sense? I feel like I want to be attached to you as a character because of who you are, and I do that best in the parts where I myself sink into the background.

Durneen

Just got evacuated from our building because a PhD student burnt some toast in the graduate room.

Ok, so I need to shift the focus. Can work on that, sure.

How do I move you into the background without losing motivation for looking for the comics?

Ah, they're letting us back in. More later.

Mahmutović

The key to the scene at the bookshop is that your character is seriously trying to do something that appears weird, and there is a motive, which you can relate, but not the entire story, just the image itself which you liked, and that's enough, because that was enough for you to go out and do this. But don't tell it as a separate story. I do like this juxtaposition between you and me, and what it does, but that can be worked into the flow as you move back and forth in time. So in my mind the story begins with your search and ends how it ends now, but the rest comes in between.

Durneen

I need to break some eggs, right? Well that can be done.

Mahmutović

yes
but i love it
you know
cant wait

Durneen

I am glad you like it though. You know I'll change whatever needs to be changed. Just wanted to send you that original draft.

Mahmutović

At first I didn't want to say anything, because I knew it was the first draft. I actually read it last night. You caught me just before I went to sleep, and I wanted to sleep on it.

Durneen

Plus this is the first personal essay I ever wrote, so need advice from the expert.

Mahmutović

But I couldn't quite fall asleep.

Durneen

But you know this essay is tricky. For so many reasons. If I cared less about it, I'd be able to write it quicker, because the words are there. I just want to get it right. "Right" means different things here. It's not just phrasing and structure.

Mahmutović

Yes, I know. But seriously, relax about it. It shows that you're not relaxed. Like you care so much about what it means you want grab me by the throat and tell me how I should feel. But the core images and textual nuances are there.

Durneen

Well … maybe not the throat … that seems kinda dangerous. I'm on it with the essay. Quick question, how much of the original comic books in septic tanks story do I want in here? Nothing? Or just a passing reference?

Mahmutović

Just a reference, just what I told you on FB when we talked about it, and not even all that.

Durneen

Ok, thanks. *disappears back into piles of paper* Oh hang on, one more question – do I want to keep the bits that are about me? From 1992.

Mahmutović

You mean the mythical discourse? Leave it aside for a while because those bits are so tied to the bits about me. I think there's a lot of good stuff there to be put in the essay.
   Timed right.

Durneen

The bits at the beginning, that were paralleled with your story. The timing is the bit I'm playing about with at the minute. I'm just trying to figure out how to introduce it (in the comic book shop) without giving too much away but without it being too vague and like the reader can't "anchor" themself somewhere.
   What I did was cut the whole of the beginning and put that to one side. So that's good, that's what you said.

Mahmutović

Well the guy needs to get that bit about the septic tank or maybe you want to keep that mysterious.

Durneen

Yes, this is the trouble, some of it doesn't make sense in the new order. But mysterious could work.

Mahmutović

Maybe not because the essay is about you chasing these things.

Durneen

I could break the scene earlier and then return to it when more information has been revealed.

Mahmutović

Play with it and let me see.

Durneen

Chasing stuff, yes. Ok, I'll think about that. Going again now . . .

Mahmutović

No worries about getting it right from the start.

Durneen

Shit! I got so into my editing that I nearly forgot to get my kids from school . . .!

Mahmutović

Me too, I almost forgot.

Durneen

We're the worst. Ok, I have *something*. Give me another half an hour or so to tidy it a bit more – but then I'll send it. It feels like it's held together by quite fragile glue, and I may have completely fucked it all up, excuse my language, but that's what drafting is for.

Oh – and I committed my cardinal sin and I switched it to 2nd person. But the distance it gave me was helpful. I realised that I needed not to "feel" in it. I thought about what you said about grabbing you by the throat and although I don't think I was (consciously) doing it to make *you* feel something, I'm fairly certain there's a distinct possibility I was trying to say that *I* felt something. So I've tried to remove that.

I don't know quite what I'm left with though. Hard to tell. Anyway, I'm just going to go back to it for a bit and then I'll send it.

Right. This isn't finished, I know that much. But it tests out the new shape. I have two versions, this one that delays the reveal until half way through and one that has it a little bit sooner. This is the one with the earlier reveal. There are mistakes in it though and unfinished sentences which I will sort, depending on which order we decide it should go in.

Mahmutović

Can you tell me what's the difference except for the reveal. I mean did that have substantial rippling effects in either draft?

Durneen

I think the later reveal prolongs the "mystery" a bit more. But that's about the only effect, I think. The first doc corrects a few sentence-level errors. Smoothes off a few sentences, that type of thing. The second doc is actually a slightly earlier draft. Read the first doc and if you don't like that order, try the second.

Mahmutović

This is much better. The voice is more even, even in the shifts. And the story more engaging now that I'm not entirely in the limelight. I got used to the second person as I kept reading, though it was a bit jarring in the beginning. You may want to be consistent in it, though, if you don't feel like using 3rd or 1st person. I do wonder what it'd look like if the voice kept changing between different persons, sliding from 1st to 3rd to 2nd to 3rd to 1st, or whatever feels best.

Regardless, I love it. It's shaping up to something really quite beautiful. Do you want any detailed input now, or do you want to let it rest for a while and then we can work on it?

It'll work so nicely with mine. God I hope we can publish them together as one two-headed piece.

Durneen

Me too. I have a feeling we'll be able to. Can I show them both to Caron now to get an objective view on how they work together? And yes please for more detailed feedback. I want to nail this tomorrow. Even since I sent you it I've worked on the beginning para which is obviously completely new and hasn't settled yet.

Mahmutović

I'm quite into this idea of unsettling. Which is why I had that thought about 1st vs 2nd vs 3rd person.

Durneen

Yes. As before, you mean. I moved it purely to allow myself to step aside for a second. Then I wondered if I liked it and wanted it to stay.

Mahmutović

Yes, but this version. I think the 2nd person is effective to 90%.

Durneen

Yes, you can't get everywhere with it, so speak.

Mahmutović

I'll have to sleep on it because it may be a matter of tweaking. It may be perfect with some tuning.

Durneen

There were some syntactical errors in changing it across though which I've been going through.

Yes, sleep on it and see what you think.

Mahmutović

Let's see, there was a bit in the 3rd person. That's when you talk about the little girl.

Durneen

Yes. some of that went awry, I noticed and I fixed it. That's distancing again too though. Perhaps I'm not getting the concept of "personal" in personal essay.

Mahmutović

I sort of liked that effect of slipping, so that's why I thought of the shifts.

Durneen

I like that you're a tough editor.

Mahmutović

What I like about the 2nd person is this Indiana Jones feel, this detective thing. So really it's justified, and honestly quite cool for a personal essay, it breaks the potential monotony of the first person, like you really don't know what you're doing but something drives you.

Durneen

Which is about the size of it. You were totally right about where to start it.

Mahmutović

Ha, not bad for a guy who thought it was smart to put his comics into a septic tank.

Durneen

Indeed.

Mahmutović

Seriously great to read so much about you.

Durneen

I'll show you the Red Book Choice story one day.

Mahmutović

Please do. I suspect if we lived on the same street we wouldn't have met.

Durneen

Probably not. I certainly wouldn't have spoken to you. That year my English teacher wrote in my report "Lucy is unwarrantably reticent." Never forgotten that. I actually saw him earlier this year in Cambridge. Told him I was a lecturer. He looked utterly shocked.

Mahmutović

Someone to contrafibulate me on my birthday.

The editing of "Everything I know about comic books* (*and what I am afraid to ask.)"

The following is the second, almost entirely reshaped draft, with the edits and comments Mahmutović made. The subsequent drafts before the final publication in *World Literature Today* contain largely minor edits, made by both Durneen, Mahmutović, and *WLT* editors. They involve fine-tuning, fact-checking, etc., while the edits below display that raw edit which is the first response to redrafting that followed a conversation on how the story might need to be rewritten. In this draft, it is obvious that Durneen has for instance followed Mahmutović's advice from the previous conversation to focus more on her own character. In a nutshell, while this draft arises in response to some of Mahmutović's comments, we can see a metamorphosis of the text not pushed or even provoked by the editor/collaborator. More and more the story is owned by Durneen and less of a response to the story about comics Mahmutović has shared with her. Some changes are explained in the footnotes. The parts in bold are Mahmutović's initial additions which may or may not have been accepted in the final version.

You're in Forbidden Planet on Burleigh Street, the new, improved store, ~~that makes a lot of promises about being~~ the world's number one for your comic book needs. This is good, because you've got a comic book need ~~and you have the feeling you might be about to put this claim to the test~~. Up until last year Forbidden Planet was a hushed place on the other side of the street; crossing the threshold was more an admission of something than an intent to purchase. But this new store is a clean well-lighted place[2] and inside, flicking through the browsers of graphic novels, you ~~have a desire~~ **want** to belong. You gaze at the high shelves, the acreage of stories

---

2   In the final stages of editing, the *WLT* editors suggested "well-lit" which Durneen rejected because "well-lighted" is a reference to her favourite Hemingway story, "A Clean and Well-Lighted Place."

~~around you~~. Some titles are familiar, most not. By 'familiar'[3] you mean the ones with characters your kids wear on their pyjamas.

Your plan is to look like you know what you're doing, because that's what Indiana Jones would do. So when you approach the desk to ask for help in tracking down early 90s Bonelli, **but not the Italian ones, the ones** from the former Yugoslavia you assume a ~~kind of~~ casual, professional air ~~as though you do this all the time~~ of a true collector. This is the way you always spend your lunch breaks. You speak this language. *No time for love, Doctor Jones.*

The assistants at the counter look at you ~~like you're mad. T~~ and their beards twitch. What's wrong with Marvel? they want to know. Wouldn't that do? But the word you have fixed on is Bonelli, so you shake your head as if you're disappointed by *their* lack of knowledge. It has to be early 90s, you say. Really, it has to be from 1992. It has to be from – you find yourself getting tangled up in the geography. The Balkans, you say in the end. You might as well have said Mars. They turn back to setting up a little diorama of Minecraft merchandise. They don't even bother to shake their heads. Try the internet, one of them says.

The internet – where everything and nothing is possible. Like you hadn't already thought of that.

In the summer of 1992 an almost-fifteen-year-old girl and her best friend went to the annual Strawberry Fair in Cambridge, England. The girl thought maybe they would ride the waltzer and pretend to drink lemon Hooch with the kids she hoped might stop giving her a hard time if she acted a little more like them. Instead, outside a dirty canvas tent she found a bucket of goldfish waiting to be transferred to the cellophane globes on the nearby Hook a Duck stand. The fish looked sad, a seething mass of orange like a solar explosion in a plastic tub. The girl and her friend looked around, picked up the unattended bucket and walked fast until they were two streets away from the fair, water surging over the bucket's lip at every step and soaking the toes of their Doc Marten 8-holes.

The girl was kind of lonely. She read a lot. Too much~~, maybe~~. The other girls in her class were pretty and were learning how to kiss the boys in the dark of the school drama theatre. The boys in her class ~~called her a nerd and~~ made vomiting sounds when they played spin the bottle and the bottle stopped on her. Somewhere around the beginning of 1992 she had decided to stop eating, as ~~if that might make a difference. As~~ if loneliness and food were ~~directly~~ connected somehow and you could fix one by rationing the other.

The girl watched Tintin on Sunday mornings and scared herself with Twilight Zone and that was as much as she knew about comic books. By the summer of 1992 she hadn't eaten anything except cabbage cooked in vegetable stock for nearly four months. She had a crush on Cyrano de Bergerac. Partly this was because of Gerard Depardieu, who hadn't yet gotten fat and started pissing in planes, but partly because she still half-believed in the existence of heroes that didn't look like heroes,

---

3   Generally, Mahmutovic cut all scare quotes.

the ones that maybe were OK about it if you got good grades and wrote poems and didn't have big boobs or straight teeth.

One time the girl's mother threw a plate of food at her **and shouted,** Why can't you just be normal? ~~the mother shouted, a~~ **A**nd she really wanted to know. The girl's father was in the business of reconnaissance. She hadn't seen him for some months. In summer 1992 she didn't actually know where he was, other than that a war in a place that was no longer Yugoslavia had taken him away.

Eventually, officially, wars come to an end. Some people get to go back home, like the girl's father. Mostly war follows you, invisibly, internally. You can make it your business to study the writing of war, but there is always the knowledge, a deep guilt in the regolith of you, that no matter how much you read you can never, actually, know. Lives converge until the moment they absolutely don't.

In the summer of 1992 or thereabouts, another thing was happening, something the girl only hears about more than two decades later, via Facebook message. A boy and his best friend pushed a wheelbarrow full of comic books into the mountains above the Bosnian city of Banja Luka to try and hide them from soldiers. Afraid that wild animals would destroy them, they came up with a different plan. Wrapping the comics in plastic bags, they lowered them into a septic tank, only to realise some time later that the bags might not be ~~so~~ shitproof ~~and the comic books not quite as safe as they believed~~. This was indeed the case. The boy used up a whole can of his mother's expensive deodorant to take away the smell ~~of shit-stained comic book paper from his attic bedroom~~. His mother wanted to kill him. His words. **[AM: This section should probably stay in the 3rd person. I like how it reads.]**

Twenty-two years later, the boy, now the girl's friend, says, I was really stupid, wasn't I?

The girl, you, **says,** ~~tells the boy, now a man, your friend Adnan, that he has to write about this — an essay on how to save comic books in time of war~~.

~~I was really stupid, wasn't I? he asks.~~
No, ~~you say,~~ and it's not entirely a lie. It's what Indiana Jones would do.
That's how little I was worried about being killed, he says. Bloody geek.
But geeks are so much cooler than nerds.
What?
Sorry. I thought that was my inside voice.

Your eldest son is a proud Doctor Who geek, and inordinately fond of that viral song "Dumb Ways to Die." He worries a lot about being killed. By solar flare, freak asteroid impact, zombie apocalypse, Ebola. You try to imagine him ~~avoiding soldiers and~~ navigating checkpoints, **hiding his stuff from soldiers,** ~~anything or even understanding that he might need to,~~ and remember how last time he made lunch for himself he used a tea strainer to drain a can of tuna fish. It's pretty unlikely the odds would be in his favour.

When ~~Adnan~~ **your friend** tells you about the comic books in the septic tank, it's like you are watching the scene ~~from somewhere far off, from above,~~ **in a snow globe, or Asimov's chronoscope,** these two kids and their wheelbarrow going up one street and down another, their frustration **growing,** ~~(and perhaps also their fear, but he doesn't mention that)~~ ~~growing~~ **[AM: I do not like brackets. They give me a sense of hiding the text as if it is not important. If it is not important, then cut it, if it is, then remove the brackets].** ~~It's like seeing the whole thing through a snow globe. Asimov's chronoscope. Vonnegut would call it slipping in time. Sometimes you just have to say these things even if they make no sense.~~

The urge to *do* something ~~is visceral, it~~ starts somewhere in your throat and rises. If you could shout down through the time vortex. If he could look up into the swirling cogs/ether/matrix to see you waving. What would you say? Throw me your comics, I'll keep them safe for you? Or – hang on, I'm coming down, let me help push the damn wheelbarrow? A **nerdy** girl, you think, ~~especially a nerdy one,~~ might have come up with a better plan than a septic tank. ~~You wonder about the things a comic book might be able to do. You wonder if a comic book has the power to change history, or what that would even mean.~~

When you said you know nothing about comic books this is ~~mostly, but~~ not entirely, true. It's just that you're not talking your Silver Surfer or Blueberry. You're definitely not talking Corto Maltese. There was a time when you and your friend Sarah were avid devotees of the *Just Seventeen* photo story, which is to say that you were romantics who had not yet experienced romance and were educating yourself on mildly erotic, post-punk tales of attraction featuring bad boys in leather jackets, which explains a lot about your respective emotional crises to come. On one occasion, planning a surreptitious photo shoot, you went to the town library in stockings and heels stolen from your mothers' wardrobes; you barely made it through the door before the librarians asked to see your borrowing cards (which you dutifully handed over) and promptly called your parents to come remove you.

That was the end of the photo shoots. But you'd caught the storytelling bug, you and Sarah, ~~like some kind of contagion,~~ the vice that Hemingway says only death can stop. You wrote and illustrated your own Choose Your Own **[AM: Not sure how to do it, but this repetition of your own is not ideal.]** Adventure strips, in first one and then a series of identical red exercise books: the destined-to-be-legendary Red Book Choice Story, which one of you still owns in an attic somewhere. The book was pretty dangerous, ~~it was fair to say~~. In it you made good stuff happen to people you liked, the teachers who were kind and didn't throw chairs. You brought to life rumours of affairs and made the cool fifth formers fall in love with you. You gave the mean kids ~~what could euphemistically be called~~ their comeuppance. It was secret, of course, until one day it wasn't. As stories went, it was a page-turner and it was gaining an underground reputation. Then ~~one girl, call her~~ Katie asked to read it. ~~You should point out here that~~ Katie was someone who took a persistent, vindictive delight in flipping up your netball skirt to reveal those blue regulation gym knickers and her narrative arc hadn't ended well. *Turn to page 48 to avenge the wrath of the schoolgirl demon.* Still, she scared you enough you didn't know how to refuse.

You sat up all night to rewrite that book, the book that had taken months to evolve organically, defiantly,~~ into a complex web of fantasies fulfilled and thwarted, ideal lives created and lived~~. When you think of it now you wonder about the way you didn't stand up for the words~~, how when faced with a test you chose to betray the truths they were supposed to expose~~. You want to believe this was what was needed to save the story (and your good-girl reputations) **[AM: Brackets again, please remove.]** – a ~~kind of~~ mild, literary collateral damage – but this is not how it feels. Now it feels something closer to cowardice. Barthes says that the book creates meaning and then that meaning creates life. If so, then the meaning you were creating was**n't shitproof** ~~fraudulent, the life a lie~~. **[AM: Just testing if this works as a connection to my story which you mention earlier.]** One thing you don't know for certain; if it came to it, if you had to, how much would you really have risked to save that book? ~~Through the reversed telescope of hindsight,~~ **In this snow globe** what you see is disappointing; two girls doing nothing but covering their steps.

~~Adnan~~ **Your friend** sends you ~~a different~~ **an** essay to proof-read, something he wrote after you met in Vienna last summer. It's ~~this one~~ about faith and forgiveness. Here you see he's ambivalent about forgiving a person who once stole his collection of Bonelli comics. He's joking, sure, but – there are those comic books again, you think. They really do mean something~~, huh?~~

You read the essay about ten times. You want to ask so many things. Bonelli, it says. *Bonelli.* You commit it to memory, which is a less abstruse way of saying it starts to haunt you. Italian. Were these the comics sunk into the septic tank and ravaged by shit and expensive deodorant? You think of that story about Hadley Hemingway, the famous one in which she catches a train to visit Ernest in Lausanne and whilst waiting at the Gare de Lyon her suitcase containing every last one of the original Nick Adams stories is stolen. You imagine the despair of knowing that there is nothing to replace the thing you have lost, an emptiness that stretches out about as long as the journey to Switzerland.

When the idea comes to you ~~– a crazy one, you see that right from the outset –~~ it comes the way anything obvious and also impossible arrives in your mind. You want to replace those ruined comic**s** ~~books~~. You know nothing about ~~comic books~~ **Bonelli, b**~~B~~ut by some chance, you work alongside magical agents and allies~~; people who actually do~~. You leave behind the sleek contemporary corridors of the university in which you teach and cross over to the Victorian halls of the Cambridge School of Art. There are geeks, collectors, and experts on graphic literature in every room, but this one seems out of even their league. Someone knows someone somewhere in Slovenia who maybe once had a thing about comic books. Will that help?

It doesn't. That's how you end up in Forbidden Planet **talking to assistants with twitchy beards who'd rather sell you the latest Spider-Man**.

But the thing about Choose Your Own Adventure is this: for every dead end, there is a way to renegotiate fate. A rope-bridge you didn't notice on page 61 leads you to safety across a gorge. As you are leaving the store, ~~the IT~~ **some** guy~~, behind the desk only to fix some system or other~~, comes up to you. He taps your sleeve

and asks, What are you after? ~~he says,~~ Dylan Dog? Martin ~~Mystère~~ **Mystery**? And immediately you understand that he heard your conversation with the **twitchy** bearded ~~assistants,~~ that by some osmotic process he appreciates the vital nature of whatever it is you're trying to do ~~better than you do yourself~~. Here is your improbable reprieve, arriving like an angel with the correct vocabulary and everything. **[AM: I really like the way you're thinking. Some details are so damn cool.]**

You tell ~~the IT guy~~ **him** you actually have no idea what you are after. It's a relief to confess it. You tell him the story of the comic**s** ~~books~~ in the septic tank. You tell him how you want to replace the shit-stained comics ~~– the lost comics~~, the ones that never made it to safety in Sweden which is where your friend ended up **after the war**~~, in a city of islands under the midnight sun, after a bus journey that took him the length of Europe~~. As you talk you realize how many gaps there are in what you know, what you're doing, but you learn this; strangers are so happy to help what they think of as a romantic (by which you mean old-school escapist, wild – and yes, crazy) notion. He pats you on the arm as if you're in need of ~~something~~. Valium, ~~maybe he's thinking~~. Okay, he says. Okay.

The ~~IT~~ guy has a friend in Sarajevo who might be able to help. He takes your email address. ~~What are the odds? you think.~~ The synchronicity buoys you up. It's like ~~another world has opened in front of you, a (secret) mission~~, **you're in** a real comic book world of mystery and clues and leads. You don't say anything to ~~Adnan~~ **your friend**. You ~~have the idea maybe you'll~~ **want to** send him the comic**s** ~~books~~ for his birthday. It occurs to you that you don't know when his birthday is. Seriously, you don't have any idea what you are doing.

What part of the human brain compels it to see everything in relative terms? It doesn't even have to be the dramatic stuff. *~~He was doing this while you were –.~~* You understand how pattern finding has a deep, biological appeal. As soon as you heard the story of the comics in the septic tank, your own history became relative. You don't mean *less*. It's just that things start to braid together in a new way; for a short time the only thing you could see, like a retina burn, was a teenage boy and his best friend sinking a plastic wrapped bundle of comic**s** ~~books~~ **[AM: I guess by now you see I prefer comics to comic books.]** into a stinking shithole while on the other side of the continent a teenage girl and her best friend, both with a labyrinth-sized crush on David Bowie, repeat-pause VHS tapes on the dance scene where the Goblin King's crotch earns a credit all to itself.

About six years ~~after the comic books were hidden in the septic tank~~ **later,** you spent a summer working as an intern in the department of Prints and Drawings in the *Musèe des Beaux Arts*, Brussels. This was the summer you learned to eat again. You didn't know it was going to work this way, but standing in the great hall looking at Brueghel's Icarus~~, the amazing boy who fell from the sky while a *ship sailed calmly on* –~~ that all turned out to be part of the recovery.

W. H. Auden wrote a poem about that painting: 'About suffering they were never wrong/the Old Masters. How well they understood/ its human position: how it takes place/while someone else is eating or opening a window.' **[AM: the**

poem should be set apart, like a block quote, you know. More effective.]
There were lots of people who saw ~~Adnan~~ **my friend** and his friend ~~Armin~~ pushing a wheelbarrow of comic books around town, but even in war, everyone has
somewhere to get to. *The sun shone as it had to*, says Auden. Perhaps one of the quiet
tragedies of being human is that everyone knows fine well how everything is relative, but also that mostly, no-one is looking. They don't see something amazing.
They see Icarus's legs disappearing into water and what they do is open a window.

Here is what starts to get braided together then; the safety of your life and the
way you were (not) eating or opening a window and the danger in his, the way he
stuck two fingers up at it, leapt over the gate of a comic book collector in inner city
Banja Luka and in defiance, entered an adventure illustrated with invincible superheroes and big-busted apocalyptic monster women, a promised land; Icarus flying
for the sun. **[AM: I get this last paragraph but even I had to think a bit.
Keep it for now and see how your friend Carol reads it, and if she gets
what is going on. This one presupposes you've read my essay.]**

A few days later you hear from the IT guy's **[AM: I like that you had that
identifying IT thing. It helps. I think I made a mistake cutting it, but the
way you introduced him was awkward so I cut that. Maybe if it was
clearer. It's not really unclear, but just a bit awkward.]** Sarajevo friend. Your
emails muddle by in a mix of pretty bad English and rusty German, which is the
best you can muster between you. He tells you that he has plenty of comics from
the late 2000s, but anything from the 90s is impossible to get hold of; those books
are like gold dust. You explain to him, in very general terms (because it's still hard
to explain to yourself, to anyone, in complex terms) **[AM: brackets again]** why
it's important. Minutes pass. Wait a moment, he ~~types~~ **writes**. Write you a new mail
**soon! [AM: I added this because this confused me. For a sec I thought it
was a chat.]**

He gets back to you later that evening. You know these are not English language?
he ~~says~~ **writes**, as if things can't proceed until this has been established. These
comics are in Croatian language.

You ask if it's possible to get them in Bosnian. His reply is a series of exclamation
and question marks and suddenly you realise a comic book is not just a comic book,
how language is not just lexis, how little you ~~understand~~ – really understand – of
that whole ~~conflict~~ **war**. ~~given you~~ **You** don't even know something fundamental
like what language your friend would read his Dylan Dog in, not for sure.

The Sarajevo guy sends you a 1998 *Marti Misterija*, in Croatian, and says it's the
best he can do, he can't get earlier. But he also has a whole bunch of Dylan Dogs
and an Alan Ford, which is his personal favourite. **[AM: Yeah, we loved Ford.
Dark humour. All characters are bad guys. Alan is not, but he's just naïve.]**
He'll send those too. Registered fast packet, he says. *Important!* You lack the real
words to show my gratitude, even though a tiny part of you is disappointed that you
couldn't get what you really wanted, whatever that was. *Hvala* doesn't quite cut it.
In English he writes that he has all (yes, all) the Martin ~~Mystère~~ **Mystery [AM:
I just think English version is best here.]** series from the beginning to a few

years ago when he stopped collecting. There are not coming so many new. . . he says and you feel the true sadness in the ellipsis. You don't ask why he stopped collecting. You are still thinking about the currency of these books. The way they might matter so much that a boy would put himself at risk to keep them safe, or that grown men would smuggle them to refugee camps. ~~They must be fucking awesome, you think~~ [AM: Ha, yes. But no, they're not. Great line.]

When they arrive, when you pore over them – in a language you can't read so you have to navigate through image alone – it is their ordinariness, the intimate, insular relationship they set up with their reader that really breaks your heart. There's a giant eyeball on the cover of the 1998 Martin ~~Mystère~~ **Mystery**. Inside, naked girls in some kind of swirling continuum. ~~Martin Mystère – Mystery in America, Misterija in Croatia, Marma Manithan Martin in South India –~~ **This MM** is an art historian, adventurer, anthropologist and collector of unusual objects. *You had me at art historian!* you want to shout. A comic book hero who is part nerd! It's not important that you understand exactly. You look at the comics and what you feel is that same thrill of discovery, of finding an entire ~~universe~~ **world** to inhabit. It's the way reading makes you feel alive; not in the way that is the opposite of death but real and present, there and nowhere else but *there*.

This much you know. The things that might change the world are the private wars people fight. The deals we make with ourselves as to how far we'd go for something we love. The something amazing is the strength and power and purpose in what those boys did up on the mountain, affording these stories of doomsdays and utopias the same status as diamonds and gold.

The war your father fought was in the air and it was public, and complicated. When your father returned from the Balkans he was a different man. Or maybe you were a different daughter and saw things you hadn't understood on his return from previous detachments; East Germany, Iraq. Lost, is the way you would describe him.

Traumatized, yes. Something your father heard in one town: a man had cut the head off his neighbour, a former friend, someone whose plants he had tended and whose dogs he had fed, and put it on a spike in his front garden. Above another town, a light attack aircraft was downed and the pilot ejected. He was found, mortally injured, by Ustaše Militia, who took him away, beat him to death and mutilated his already wounded body.

~~Adnan writes to you one day about an old television monologue, the story of a peasant who goes to Austria to work. The peasant meets this man who tells him there's no such country as Bosnia.~~

~~No matter what the narrator says, Adnan writes, the man stubbornly refuses all arguments, so the narrator gets so pissed he leaves the good life and goes back to his village out of spite. It's so funny.~~

~~What happens when he gets back to his village? you ask, trying to imagine how it is funny when it sounds so sad.~~

~~The story ends. He walks down the hill, heavily gesticulating. Repeating the words angrily, 'and he tells ME there's no Bosnia.'~~ [AM: I do like this, but it doesn't work here. I'd cut it all.]

A week or so later your Sarajevo contact emails out of the blue to say he's been thinking. He might have something for you. He's actually got pretty much every comic out there, but he won't sell. What he will do is scan them and put some on DVD. Any ones you like. There is something in this offer, this considered, delayed response, the desire to help flashed through with the desire to preserve the integrity of his collection at all costs, that makes you feel sad and simultaneously connected to something. Such generosity amongst an underground network of geeks. Your only tangible experience of Bosnia is this, a chain of comic books forming a chain out across, under, around Europe and the way those who know will go out of their way to restore the gaps in the narrative.

Once a semester you and your colleague Caron host an Open Mic Poetry night where you encourage your students to read and perform their own work. They are all afraid of poetry, but they like the camaraderie, the free wine and the craic. You stand at the front of the lecture hall backlit by a PowerPoint that reads: *Words Have Power*. Words are smuggled from concentration camps, you tell them, through border posts, over mountains. Words are swallowed and remembered and burned into us in order that they survive. This is why we do what we do. This is why we write. This is why we read. Sometimes you wonder if this means anything to twenty-first-century teenagers whose biggest concerns involve thigh gaps and who their favourite celebrity is sleeping with. Then someone stands up, the quiet kid at the back who hasn't spoken yet, and reads about how his father is in prison for murdering his brother and you realise that it's not just the words that survive; we risk everything for them so that the strongest parts of ourselves will too.

That's how little ~~he~~ I was afraid of being killed. **[AM: my words, right?]**

You're not sure if you believe ~~Adnan~~ **him** when he says this. But then, you know this to be true enough: on the only occasion you can say you were truly in grave and immediate danger of dying, you were ~~surprisingly,~~ pathologically, practical. Half-mad with pain and morphine, you made arrangements with the theatre nurse, who humoured you by taking real notes, to cover your postgraduate dissertation supervision for a week. You told the anaesthetist that under no circumstances was he to have an argument with the surgeon over the afore-mentioned nurse if you went into VF, the way they did on the hospital shows. It's ok, he said, we're all happily married here. Then he pressed down on your windpipe to stop your stomach contents entering your lungs and put you under/shut you up. **[AM: pick one]** You had no intention of ~~actually~~ dying, although the odds at the time were relatively high. You didn't even know what VF meant. What you're really saying is that maybe in the face of ~~true~~ danger, we assume a hero's level of pragmatism, a clear ability to compartmentalise what is being risked away from what is needed, what is desired. It's possible this qualifies as a superpower~~, awesome in the real sense of the word; life-affirming~~.

You don't write back straight away to ~~the IT guy's friend in~~ Sarajevo **guy**. You're not quite sure what you'd be asking for. A DVD doesn't seem quite the same somehow. It's the tangible object, the restoration – the sheer materiality of ~~the~~ **your** quest – that has been driving you, the book nerd's fantasy of the longed-for manuscript pressed into the outstretched hand. If you could travel to the afterlife and present

Hemingway with a DVD of those stories from the suitcase stolen at the Gare de Lyon, you're pretty sure he would throw a daiquiri in your face.

The weather is turning cold here. One day ~~Adnan~~ **your friend** messages to tell you ~~his~~ **he wrote an** essay~~, the real essay~~ on how to save comic books in time of war~~, is finished.~~ **He did it because you told him to. There's more to the story than what's in your snow globe. More than the wheelbarrow and the septic tank.**

You're about to give an undergraduate writing class on constructing character. You're planning to do an exercise that draws on Tim O'Brien's story "The Things They Carried," **because** you want your students to leave behind the trappings of their own autobiographies, just for a moment. Instead, at the very last minute, you ditch the schedule and tell them the true story of the boy who hid his comics in the septic tank. ~~'The things we risk our life for'.~~ You watch your students' faces change as you talk. ~~You have their complete attention, all of them, e~~Even the two at the back who have been talking about the work they haven't done for their Renaissance Drama module **are listening to you.** ~~Everyone sits quietly with~~ The sharp winter light **is** streaming through the windows.

Even now you have not told ~~Adnan~~ **your friend** what you've been doing. Part of you is a little embarrassed. You experience what you come to think of as a distant cousin of survivor's guilt, but it's a superlative guilt that recycles and reactivates itself, guilty twice over – once for the simple fact that you didn't suffer his suffering, and again for its own fraudulent act of existing; this isn't even authentic, you survived nothing; it's survivor's guilt by proxy. ~~Your students are obsessed by the idea of ouroboros, something chasing its own tail.~~ Maybe this is your ouroboros come to get you. Damn it.

In your tea break, you go back to your stuffy office and write your friend the pathetic story of how you tried and failed to hunt down ~~the~~ **his** comic~~s~~ ~~books that may or may not have been destroyed during, or after, their meeting with the septic tank.~~ You hesitate, just for a moment, before pressing *send*. You're worried he will think badly of you, that he will think you stupid for believing that replacing a comic book might heal the other kinds of wound that war leaves a person with, the ones your friendship is too new, too distant to let you see, but the ones his fun stories about sad refugees tell you exist. Or worse, that he will know you have only an outsider's perspective and will think you are romanticising something, appropriating what you're not entitled to.

What he really wanted back then, now, both, was to be a comic book hero. You think about the ways to tell him he kind of already is.

Here is one way.

Tell him about the night the lonely girl, now a grown woman, hears the story of the comic~~s~~ ~~books~~ for the first time. How she goes to sleep restless. How it feels as though her heart has been cut out, but in the morning – ~~like the plant in the desert found by Ondaatje's English Patient~~ – she will wake to find it full and the restlessness renewed. Tell him how at first she thinks it's a kind of melancholia, but ~~it's not,~~ it's stranger and stronger than that. It is a teenage girl's breathless admiration for a teenage boy's ~~valiant~~ bravado, combined with a mother's fear that any terrible thing that has ever happened to a child will now or in the future happen to her child. [**AM: Damn**] It is the concrete distillation of an abstract truth; that all the world's dark ugliness has never yet been able to stop that thing Nadine Gordimer calls the firefly flash of real life.

Tell him how that night the girl checked in on her son, as she does every night. How she saw in sleep little visible sign of the man he was slowly becoming. How it was hard not to compare him to the boy in the attic room **in Bosnia**, dreaming about his comics as they drift through raw sewage in their dark, plastic wombs. A little older than her son is now, true, but still a boy, just, whatever he'd probably say.

Don't tell him how she would cry for those shitty comic books she can't smell, because he wasn't crying over them and they were his comics. Explain that you will not forget this story of how once, two boys in Banja Luka did something brave and stupid and kind of miraculous. Miracles aren't always obvious. Miracles happen when someone is closing a window, or walking dully along. When it comes to it, really all you have to give is a story of a bungled comic book rescue, ~~not the book itself~~ – not the object restored – and it is a very small thing. Give it. You may as well.

~~This is what you are saying: now you understand that nothing beats reading comics in wartime anyway.~~ [**AM: this copies my ending too much so I cut it. I want your ending to be yours.**]

Conversation between Lucy Durneen, Adnan Mahmutović, and Friðrik Sólnes Jónsson

Since both Durneen and Mahmutović are the authors of this present volume, Jónsson was asked to look through the process of drafting and editing and engage in a discussion with them.

Jónsson

Lucy, in your case, we can follow the evolution of the essay from the very first, raw draft, until the published version. The differences in narrative style and flow, tone, and other aspects of craft, are great, and yet I find that the core remains the same. It becomes clearer and clearer, but it does not change with the change of form. Rather, the process of redrafting and editing becomes an attempt to find the right form for the story that is already there. I wonder, how many separate drafts were there? In the most general terms, what drove the development of the essay from the first draft to the finished version? Reader comments? Your own revisions? The editor's demands?

Durneen

Actually, I cannot remember how many individual drafts there were (if we are going to think of separate drafts as being like specific stations on the route to the finished piece), but I think of there being three key stages in terms of editing, which is what we display here in this book. First there was the initial draft, which was written in the first person and was in many ways just for me, to externalize my own experience, and to order and make sense of it. I never really imagined it being for public consumption. This was raw and held together by a framework that drew on the stages of Joseph Campbell's monomyth, as a means of trying to rein in what was quite a complex narrative, chronologically. The second draft was more mindful of its relationship to Adnan's original piece, and shifted into second person to enable a certain level of distance that I felt I needed. This was the stage at which Adnan and I worked most closely and consciously on actively changing and shaping the essay. And then there was the final draft that made it into print with *World Literature Today*.

To generalise, the most significant of those changes, the perspective shift, was driven by – although I see this most clearly in hindsight – a need to retreat a little from the material. That is to say, it was a personal essay that was also something of a re-telling of someone else's story, and a wider reflection on the power of words, and I think Adnan said at one point was it was "grabbing him by the throat," which of course was not at all the effect I was aiming for. And more than that, I was conscious of that thing Celia Hunt calls "page-fright," that fear of seeing oneself, in unexpurgated ugliness and foolishness, right there in front of you, and what became evident to me was that it would be necessary to hide a little in order to be able to control the story I was trying to tell.

Jónsson

In the conversation, you tell Adnan that his story about the comics in the septic tank really stuck with you. How did this project come about? And how did you (both) discover that the year 1992, comics, and war were topics that together had a special significance for both of you, in a way connected you, and could be developed into a joint project?

Durneen

Even though I love the finished piece so much, I still do not feel I can truly communicate the impact of that first moment of hearing about the comics in the septic tank. How I was knocked flat by the craziness of what these two boys had done out there in the mountains, the simplicity of their response to the war around them. How I loved, and was in awe of, their bravery. There is a moment in William Styron's novel *Sophie's Choice* where Stingo thinks about what he was doing while Sophie was standing on the station ramp at Auschwitz and, as I recall, he concludes that he was probably doing something as banal as eating a banana. The night we talked about it, I was thinking – so what was I doing while Adnan was packing comics into the septic tank? My father was on long-term RAF detachment in the Balkans, I was anorexic and trying to figure out who I was, as a girl, as a writer. Much of my loneliness was caused by the idea of being a nerd, which was NOT cool back in 1992, and by the fear my father would not return from this new war whose origins

I barely felt I understood. Even as I was trying to track down these comics to be able to replace them for an adult Adnan who had probably long stopped mourning their loss, I realized I was also addressing some deeper wounds of my own, and ones that I felt I could reveal to him (in the spirit of 'I'll show you my pain if you show me yours'). So, for me, this piece is also about friendship, and the places in which we find acceptance of ourselves, the places we can be uncensored, as much as it is about comics, war, or anything that happened in 1992.

Mahmutović

It started by me feeling that Lucy was the kind of friend who I could tell a story like that and not feel she'd make fun of me. The reaction was not only acceptance but admiration too, which I did not expect, so I felt brave enough to come out of the closet as a geek. The rest happened organically as we had a true transnational exchange, an exchange colored by understanding and acceptance and nothing else.

Jónsson

How and when did *World Literature Today* become involved?

Mahmutović

I had earlier published in *WLT*, which in my view is one of the best magazines in the world. Their dedication to world literature is pure. They seek to make borders more porous and show how our love of literature makes us connect in the most incredible ways. I thought they would appreciate a story like this, which does everything they stand for. And they did.

Jónsson

How involved was *WLT* as a publisher? Did they make their own suggestions regarding form, content, word count etc., or place any other demands or constraints on the project?

Durneen

No constraints. In fact, they published the two essays even though they are four times longer than what they usually allow. We worked on some smaller edits, and the major work was done in terms of images from comics mentioned in the essays. They used a number of cool pictures, and created a stunning design in both the print and the online version (which included a video of us reading our pieces). I made last-minute changes as I realized that the *Martin Mystery* comic I had found was in fact a reissue, not the 1998 original. I was gutted. But Michelle at *WLT* was very accommodating in terms of allowing me to amend a paragraph to reflect this lost in translation moment – more than that, extremely sensitive, I thought, to that sense that a piece is never truly finished and continues to respond to the circumstances that generated it in the first place. I was lucky to have the creative freedom there right up to the wire.

Jónsson

Are you happy with the finished product? Any regrets or reservations?

Durneen

No regrets. I am more proud of this piece – the finished essay *duet* – than perhaps anything else I've ever written. I am also consistently surprised at the power of the two pieces in tandem, and it is my only piece that, even two years after the point of writing, still has the ability to evoke in me the raw emotion of the thing that prompted me to write in the first place. For this reason, I know that we were successful in finding the right articulation for the story, the right balance between personal essay and a broader dialogue with the themes raised in Adnan's original. It *was* difficult, it *was* painful, but I absolutely trusted Adnan's edits were taking the piece in the most appropriate direction with every suggested move.

That said, I still wonder a little about the second person perspective, if in some ways it was not another act of literary cowardice on my part. For the BBC Radio adaptation, we worked in first person throughout, to really create that sense of an asynchronous dialogue, across time, across a continent, and it makes me think that there might have been more to explore on that front. But the radio piece came 18 months on. I was bolder then. I had become accustomed to the story being in the public domain and the need to use the narrative as a kind of cloaking device was less acute.

Mahmutović

I was more than happy with the final version. I felt I was in a difficult situation since I had a few roles in the process. The first, and most important, role was being the partial subject of Lucy's essay. While my own piece was local, or vernacular, solely focused on my own experience, Lucy's story was transnational from the start. Hers was a unique hybrid of a personal essay and a response to someone else's (hi)story. That is utterly unusual and when they were put together Lucy's text had a more direct address to mine while mine had only an implicit conversation with hers. Given all this, and the fact we were good friends, it was immensely difficult for me to approach it as a critic and editor. Some of my feedback and editorial input was most definitely affected by the very core and the *raison d'être* of Lucy's essay. This is why I pushed her to push me out of the story, including the erasure of my name. I was OK being a trigger for her own story but it felt like she was devaluing her own history which is something I have always been sensitive to, as a refugee trying to assert my own voice in different countries and in different languages. For me it was essential that she owned and valued her history. When we later worked on the radio piece which was even more of a dialogue, we pushed this sense of the stories touching mainly through coincidence and less in terms of pure, direct response. This was one of the best writing experiences I ever had.

Jónsson

I want to ask straight out if you agreed with all his suggestions? Were there any especially difficult concessions?

Durneen

Something I really value in my writing-editing relationship with Adnan is that I never really have to explain to him what I am trying to do with a piece, and so the process of editing becomes, as you noticed yourself, more about making the real story visible, rather than a sense of *correcting* it. For me this is not a common experience. The level of trust it requires is immense. I read over our Facebook conversations regarding the piece and I am amazed at how . . . incomplete . . . we are in terms of editorial suggestions, how often the initial suggestions lack actual detail – it is like a dancer nodding at her partner to indicate the move to come; you just know what you are supposed to do next. So what is happening here is that he is giving me the means to see more acutely the thing that I am trying to do. In a way, his suggestions were really things that instinctively I understood I had to do but had not identified in concrete terms. To answer your question, it also meant that there were no real concessions. Where bigger changes needed to be made, at some level I had already acknowledged there was an issue to be resolved there.

Jónsson

Do you feel that the finished product reflects your own style of writing? Was there anything in particular you fought for and won? Anything in particular you fought for and lost?

Durneen

We do not fight. As I said before, this is not how we work. It is not like one of those famous, and stereotyped relationships where the editor is the bad guy who compromises the artist's vision. The piece grew quite organically out of conversations rather than a conscious attempt to merge two styles into one, and actually I think there is something about the way Adnan and I write that is at one and the same time complementary and distinct, so it never felt as though I was compromising anything during the editing process. One of the best suggestions Adnan made – the most necessary – was to make him *sink into the background* as a presence in my story, and I think that allowed for a kind of exchange, for my Self (writing Self/remembered Self) to step forward and assert itself a little more.

Jónsson

Both of you are lecturers in creative writing and editing with years of education and experience in the field. I imagine you both have a shared vocabulary for discussing a text but also some individually fully formed ideas regarding how a text should look. How did this affect your project? Did it help? Are you, simply put, as good at taking criticism as you are at giving it?

Durneen

I am not after flattery when it comes to feedback, and I think Adnan recognizes that. His feedback is not unduly harsh, but it does not usually sugar the pill either. This is possible in part because of our underlying friendship. You do develop your own codes, your own vocabulary of feedback, which is not quite the same as that which either of us would use in the classroom. He sees what needs to be done and because I respect him as a writer as well as an editor I am not worried about giving the suggestions a go. Our aesthetic sensibilities are pretty much in line. More often than not, doing so either turns out to be the correct move, or an alternative reveals itself during the process. It makes me a more attentive drafter and pushes my writing harder, full stop.

Mahmutović

I love to get, and to give tough critique but I was afraid of giving one to Lucy in the beginning when her essay was fresh because it felt so personal, so much an expression of her friendship, and I was not sure how that affected my critical mind. At the same time, I could not take off my teacher/editor hat and had lots of thoughts, but I gave them only after I was sure she wanted them.

Jónsson

Seeing as the two pieces were published head to head, or as two pieces complementing one another to form one whole, there is a degree of uniformity between the texts in terms of subject matter as well as the metafictional aspect. Did you work towards uniformity in style, voice or any other way? How?

Durneen

No, in fact it was very important that the pieces retained their individual voices. In my head I had this notion, always, running underneath the writing process, of this nerdy, almost-15-year-old English girl breathless with admiration, talking to this slightly older, cooler, Bosnian geek (to a nerd, *cool geek* is not an oxymoron) who had no idea she existed. Although my piece is ultimately filtered through my adult self, I wanted to retain that sense of two adolescent worlds touching but not quite merging. Our experiences mirrored each other in these surprisingly concrete ways, but of course they were never shared. We joked one time that if we had lived on the same street back then we probably would not have spoken to each other, which actually needed to be, if not explicitly so, evident in the structure and style of the piece itself.

Mahmutović

Our essays are different in style, but yes, they have a number of points where they connect and disconnect. There was never an attempt to make them closer than they were by virtue of shared experiences and feelings. All points of connection are natural, so to speak, and not a matter of narrative design. When we worked on the radio adaptation for BBC Radio 4, we had to emphasize such connections, but we tried not to find more. Instead, we relied on the ones we already had and just utilized that.

Jónsson

Considering that Adnan's piece had already been drafted when the idea of a companion piece came about, how did it affect your creative process? Did it help it along or constrain the writing?

Durneen

I felt a certain urgency to write my piece. I had something I needed to say in response to Adnan's own essay, something which I'd only partially told him at the time he shared the comics story, and the essay was the means of doing that. More than admiration but this deep, almost maternal desire to have made the outcome of that story somehow different. I wanted him to know I understood what it felt like to be a geek.

Jónsson

I realize that collaboration on texts is not a new thing (examples are Hardt & Negri, Deleuze & Guattari), but in your case the Facebook Messenger seems to have facilitated a closer and more personal collaboration. There is a very modern, technological aspect to your project. Is this correct and does this perhaps mean that we will see more of similar projects in future? Can you imagine your project (or a similar project) coming into fruition before Facebook, through email, letters, telephone calls and meeting in person?

Durneen

If you look back over the conversations, but even further back to the original sharing of the comics story, they are often written in little snatched moments of time, between teaching, or doing other things with our families, and that's something that Facebook offers – immediacy (so you can respond to a train of thought quickly), informality, (so you do not have to write more than a line at a time if that's all you have time or inclination for) but also a kind of intimacy paradoxically created by distance (so you can say things you might not in someone's physical presence). Even our editing process could be done on the hoof – while waiting in line for coffee sometimes, as I recall. I think that is an interesting development in the practice of editing – the immediacy of media like FB keeps the vitality of a project alive during that potentially dry stage of changes where, previously, the time elapsed in passing drafts back and forth by email or even hard copy might risk the real purpose of the edits being forgotten, or their significance reduced.

Jónsson

I want to look at some specific edits. Let me begin with the fact that Mahmutović keeps objecting to your use of brackets. He writes: "I do not like brackets. They give me a sense of hiding the text as if it is not important. If it is not important, then cut it, if it is, then remove the brackets." Here he explains it, and it makes sense in terms of bringing you out of hiding so to speak, but in the next instance he very much tells you to cut them. The brackets are gone in the published version, but I wonder if you share his view generally or was it just in this story that you felt he was right?

Durneen

I felt he was right. He usually is. The way he articulated it made it abundantly clear that I had to make a decision about what was being buried in parenthesis, and confront why it was I was using them so much. In this case, I realized that it wasn't so much that the text wasn't important but that I needed to work harder to unravel certain threads of thought – it wasn't just about deleting the brackets themselves but reconsidering and restructuring the ideas I was trying to contain inside them. Another thing he's taught me is to abandon that all-too-common tripartite structure of description – three adjectives, three metaphors instead of one. *Pick the one that works best and just use that*, he's told me. In this he is also right. Stop hedging your bets over description. Most editing boils down this really – standing by your words or accepting that they're redundant in some way, and this can be hard, especially for relatively inexperienced writers. We all know we're supposed to kill our darlings, but it's trickier to know how to dispose of them afterwards, or how to fill the gaps they leave behind.

Jónsson

The form and the structure became an issue from the very first moments in your conversation. Adnan's first specific reaction was to the opening. He asks you to own your narrative: "the story may be centering around this thing I told you, but it's about you. I'd begin with the scene when you're going to the store, because it shows so much about your character, and then unfold. Linearity takes away something from the entire thing. Imagine that snow globe and the story is you drifting in and out of it, reaching in and pulling out. I feel like I want to be attached to you as a character because of who you are, and I do that best in the parts where I myself sink into the background." There is this metaphor of the snow globe which allows you to see the entire thing developing, and you as the narrator then decide which points of entry you are going to make, because each entry is a sort of crack in the glass dome.

Durneen

The image of the snow globe was something that came up quite organically in the process of writing the first draft, and it was an integral part of that narrative. The only way I could really describe the way the story of the septic tank made me feel was with this metaphor, of distance, watching something that I couldn't change, but merely observe, the way we do the miniature world trapped inside the dome. But actually, this came to represent something of the editing process itself. The way Adnan described the snow globe created an organising principle. The globe acted as a concrete symbol of that distancing process – that restoration of my story, rather than re-telling Adnan's, as the narrative's focus. We kept returning to it – an example of the kind of private vocabulary we were speaking of earlier – to shape the next major draft. It seemed to say a lot about the way we might (in general) enter a story, not just in terms of finding the right voice, but the right location, the right crack from the personal into something more universally compelling. It also reinforced the limitations of what I was doing in my half of the duet – part of what I was trying to express was the agony, really, of not being able to get inside that dome and change things. Every time I felt myself trying to step too close to Adnan's story, the snow globe metaphor would come back out and course-correct.

Jónsson

I asked you earlier about style and negotiations, winning or losing fights, and the specific thing I now remember is related to the image of the snow globe, which returns in the end of your essay. It struck me that Mahmutović added a sentence: "One day ~~Adnan~~ **your friend** messages to tell you ~~his~~ **he wrote an** essay~~, the real essay~~ on how to save comic books in time of war~~, is finished~~. **He did it because you told him to. There's more to the story than what's in your snow globe. More than the wheelbarrow and the septic tank.**" I understand how the recurring image creates a connection over space and time, a connection that arises despite the fact there is no synchronic connection, but I wonder about the insertion itself. Adding as much as three sentences is unusual. Here he seems to take the liberty, very much asserting that he is attuned to your writing so he could do that.

Durneen

He is. It's unusual, and I don't have that kind of writing relationship with anyone else (it might offend me, even, with another partner) but this is very deep-rooted collaboration – to return to the metaphor of dancing, a kind of textual milonga, maybe. The smallest of cues can indicate where to move next. The partnership is dependent on the ability to interpret intention and then to perform it, externalize it. The process of writing these essays felt like this. And I do think that some ideas hide from us, some crucial parts of the story we're trying to tell – maybe because we're uncertain of them, ashamed or embarrassed even, or simply in a kind of denial, and a second pair of eyes reading the text can see those omissions in a way that we ourselves, faces pressed right up against the glass of the narrative, can't. It's like someone instantly finding your car keys when you've spent an hour looking.

Jónsson

Speaking of connections, there is a place in the edit where Mahmutović inserts the word "shitproof," which is a direct reference to his story, that segment when he packs the comics and sinks them into a septic tank, while suspecting the bags were not shitproof. He comments: "Just testing if this works as a connection to my story which you mention earlier." Since he has been pushing you to make fewer references to his essay, how does this make sense? This same word is used in your radio adaptation for BBC Radio 4. In contrast, in another place, where you retell the part of him jumping over a fence in search for comics, he comments: "I get this last paragraph but even I had to think a bit. Keep it for now and see how your friend Caron reads it, and if she gets what is going on. This one presupposes you've read my essay." Then we can see Mahmutović cut your ending with the following comment: "~~This is what you are saying: now you understand that nothing beats reading comics in wartime anyway.~~ **[AM: this copies my ending too much so I cut it. I want your ending to be yours.]**" So "shitproof" is acceptable but not the rest. How do you determine what works and what does not? Is it pure instinct or is there some logic to it?

Durneen

"Shitproof" makes sense because Adnan's looking for synchronic connections, subtler in that they work through a kind of reflex recognition in the reader – the second and third examples are more a direct mirroring of his words, a more heavy-handed way of reminding the reader that this story has been told in another way elsewhere. Adnan's a very delicate storyteller in that sense, whereas perhaps I (until now) haven't always trusted enough in the reader picking up on such small nods and gestures. But instinctively I understood it was the right approach. The two essays had to stand alone and ideally could be read in either order, but equally they were not mutually exclusive; while Adnan's essay doesn't need a "reason" to be written, mine exists as a response to his story: *I am because you are*. I'd never written this way before, so it required new strategies in terms of narrative structure and internal logic. This kind of strategizing is, for me, one of the most invaluable aspects of a writing-editing relationship.

Jónsson

Thank you for the conversation and for sharing your work.

INDEX

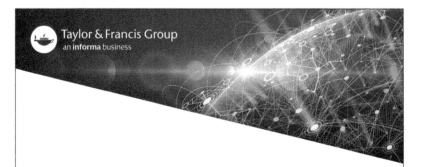